Letter from the P_____
Amanda Klenner

I could eat a whole clove of roasted garlic in one sitting and be happy as a clam – even if I would smell like garlic for a week. Thankfully my husband doesn't mind the garlic smell as he is used to me smelling like a well-herbed Italian meal. Just think, by eating a meal with rosemary, basil, garlic, marjoram, and oregano, not only am I enjoying an amazing meal, but I am also enjoying the health benefits of all of these herbs in one sitting without tinctures, salves, infusions, decoctions or other time consuming herbal preparations. Have a cold? Have some well herbed chicken soup – a delicious dose of medicinal herbs in one sitting and the kids don't even know they have taken their "medicine."

You will notice in this issue we have a ton of recipes, and few specific indications of garlic. This is because eating your way to good health can treat pretty much every issue we discuss in the Materia Medica.

Not only is garlic delicious and easy to add to just about any savory recipe, making it an easy addition to most meals, it is also a medicinal gold mine. Its antibiotic properties are what people focus on most, but it is also a well-known cardio protector and hepatoprotective, making it a tonic that can be enjoyed daily with great health benefits.

We include garlic in our meals at least once a day, but when my husband was diagnosed with high blood pressure we decided to add Kyolic garlic capsules to his daily routine. Large amounts of fresh garlic give him indigestion so, in this case, supplementing with the fresh herb was not an option for him. Kyolic is one brand (of many) that makes scent-free garlic capsules that do not cause the unwanted indigestion some get from fresh garlic. This way, he gets the health benefits of garlic without the unwanted side effects, which is nice.

We love garlic, as you can tell, and hope after this issue you will too. Enjoy!

- *Amanda*

Table of Contents

Garlic Herbal Monograph	3
Garlic Flower Essence	8
Garlic History and Mythology	10
Garlic for Winter Illness	**14**
Garlic for Ears	**18**
Garlic in the Kitchen: A Powerful Herbal Ally	**25**
Heart Healthy Garlic	**34**
Garlic is as Good as Ten Mothers!	37
Get the Garlic In	**42**
Kitchen Medicine: Garlic (*Allium sativa*)	**50**
Glossary of Herbalism	**57**
Disclaimer	**65**

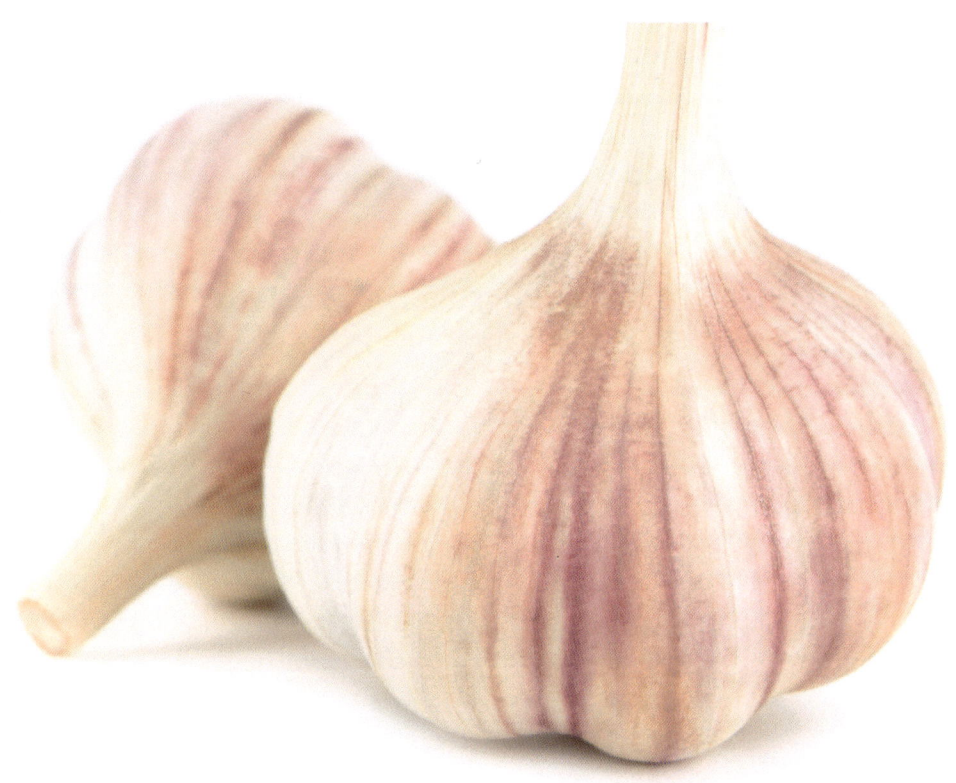

Garlic Herbal Monograph
Nina Katz

Common Name: Garlic

Latin Name: *Allium sativum*

Family: Amaryllidaceae

Other Names: the stinking rose

ACTIONS:

anti-bacterial, anti-viral, anti-fungal, anti-protozoal, immunostimulant, antineoplastic, cardiotonic, anticoagulant, stomachic, hair tonic, skin tonic

Topically: anti-bacterial, anti-viral, anti-fungal, insect repellant, anti-septic

Chemical Constituents: sulfur compounds (over 33!), amino acids (arginine, glutaminic acid, glutamine, leucine, lysine, valine, aspartic acid, tryptophan, and others that vary with the variety of garlic), calcium, choline, vitamins C and A, phosphorus, potassium,

magnesium, sodium selenium, essential oils, omega-6 and omega 3 fatty acids

Whether "Phew" or "Ahhh," reactions toward garlic are often passionate. The "stinking rose" has lovers and detractors, but few are indifferent to its odor and flavor. Personally, I think it deserves its own place in the food pyramid. As a popular ingredient in cooking, it has gained more notice for its medicinal qualities than many medicinal herbs.

Many people know of garlic as an immune stimulant that helps fight off colds and flus, and indeed, it is a potent anti-viral, anti-bacterial, and anti-fungal agent. Folk traditions about its use abound. Known as the "Russian antibiotic," garlic has adherents the world over, including among scientific researchers.

Garlic has traditionally been regarded as a respiratory remedy. In Traditional Chinese Medicine, white colored foods are associated with the lungs. It has been used for asthma, bronchitis, and pneumonia. Garlic infused in boiled, unpasteurized, fresh milk is a traditional Russian remedy for whooping cough.

Research has demonstrated that raw garlic extracts can inhibit all kinds of bacteria, including E-Coli and both gram-positive and gram-negative *Staphylococcus* bacteria.

Garlic's potent protective powers and high sulfur content have inspired some research into its use in both prevention and treatment of cancer. Medical literature mentions garlic for preventing and treating colorectal, lung, breast, prostate, brain, liver, skin, and stomach cancers, but most studies have focused on colorectal, stomach, and lung. Studies show that colorectal and stomach cancer arises less often among those who down large quantities of garlic (either raw or cooked) regularly than among those who don't; risk of colorectal cancer was reduced by 30%. Similarly, high intake of raw garlic seems to offer some protection against lung cancer to smokers and to those restaurant workers and others exposed to fumes from cooking oils heated to high temperature. In addition, a study of people with colorectal cancer reported a 29% reduction in both the size and the number of lesions among those taking an aged garlic extract.

Garlic is an excellent ally for the heart. It reduces blood pressure, particularly in people with elevated blood pressure, so it remains safe for those with low blood pressure. It relaxes the blood vessels, and may also lower cholesterol; studies conflict about this, but there is a clear correlation between heart health and garlic consumption. Garlic also acts as an anti-coagulant, reducing the risk of stroke by preventing excessive blood clotting. Studies conflict about how effective it is at lowering cholesterol.

Garlic also reduces the blood sugar level, and so is helpful in diabetes.

While some people find garlic a challenge to digest, others consider it a digestive aid. It is used specifically in the treatment of diarrhea and infant colic. Garlic aids in the production of digestive enzymes, and also helps to eliminate intestinal parasites. As an anti-bacterial, it helps the immune system fight off the bacteria that lead to ulcers.

Garlic is most potent when raw, fresh, and crushed and when not heated above room temperature; some of its sulfur compounds and enzymes are released only when crushed or cut, and some break down from heat, although they are fairly stable at room temperature. Garlic is also an ingredient in Fire Cider, the wonderful medicinal vinegar introduced by Rosemary Gladstar and commonly prepared with one crushed head of garlic, one chopped onion, a few inches each of ginger and horseradish, and a chili pepper or two, macerated in apple cider for a month, and then served to taste, neat or with water, sometimes with honey. Crushed garlic may also be infused in honey for a syrup. I also like to fill a small mason jar completely with crushed garlic and pour olive oil over it to use as a spread. Water-based preparations remain fully effective for up to 48 hours.

Topical Uses

Ukrainian schoolchildren were traditionally sent to school with garlic necklaces for protection during the flu season. Perhaps this is the origin of garlic's reputation for keeping away vampires? Garlic slices in the sock, like cloves worn around the neck, really do enhance immunity and protect against infection, because when the garlic rests against the skin, some is absorbed. Some people find that if they wear garlic in their socks, their breath soon takes on the familiar aroma.

Whether or not it is effective against vampires, garlic does repel mosquitos and a variety of other insects, including ticks. Eating garlic may suffice to protect someone whom the bugs find mildly attractive, but if you're one of their favorites, then please use garlic topically as well. A slice in the shoe or sock, some garlic oil, tincture, or liniment applied topically should do the trick.

Garlic also works topically as an anti-fungal for local fungal and yeast infections. Women sometimes make a garlic tampon to address yeast. As an anti-bacterial, it is used for trichomoniasis as well. If you are doing this, please make sure to remove it afterwards! Most people won't experience burning if they don't slice the garlic, but some women prefer to leave it wrapped in its skin. Make sure the skin is reasonably clean and doesn't have fertilizer on it!

Garlic is also used externally for treating warts, psoriasis, pruritus, and for softening calluses. Both internal and external use of garlic can help with joint pains, including those caused by both osteoarthritis and rheumatoid. It helps with muscle pains as well. Externally, the garlic is applied directly to the joints as a liniment, vinegar, or oil. A heated garlic poultice works as well.

One of the most famous topical uses of garlic is for ear infections. In America, the standard herbal treatment is to dropper some garlic-mullein oil into the ear, holding the head at a tilt for a while so that it can drip into the inner ear. (Do not put it, or anything else, into the inner ear directly!!) Garlic oil or mullein oil solo will do the job as well. In Russia, the clove, or a piece of the clove, is inserted into the outer ear and allowed to permeate slowly.

Garlic has recently become popular for hair and scalp conditioning and shampooing. Its nutritional profile promotes hair growth, but it may also address some of the underlying issues in baldness, which can be caused by immune deficiency, fungal infections, or nutritional deficiencies. Garlic can help with dandruff if it is caused by either dermatitis or fungal infections, and it is also said to prevent split ends. The commercial garlic shampoos do not have a garlicky smell. For a homemade garlic shampoo, try including parsley and perhaps essential oils along with the garlic oil, and then report back to the NLM forum.

Additionally, cilantro, parsley, cloves, fennel, and cinnamon can all help prevent garlic from perfuming the breath.

Contraindications

Some people experience digestive distress from garlic.

Do not take garlic within seven days of surgery as it does have blood thinning qualities. Do not take in medicinal doses with blood thinning drugs or if you have a blood clotting disorder.

When used topically as a poultice, garlic has been known to cause skin redness and irritation. If this happens discontinue its use in this way.

Reference

- http://cancerpreventionresearch.aacrjournals.org/content/6/7/711.abstract
- http://www.ncbi.nlm.nih.gov/pubmed/11238811
- http://www.ncbi.nlm.nih.gov/pubmed/17885009
- Al-Astal, Zakaria Y., "Effect Of Storage And Temperature Of Aqueous Garlic Extract On The Growth Of Certain Pathogenic Bacteria," Journal of Al Azhar University-Gaza 2003,Vol. 6, 2 P.11-20
- http://www.separationsnow.com/details/ezine/sepspec11539ezine/New-technique-uncovers-Garlic-and-broccoli-amino-acids.html?tzcheck=1
- http://phys.org/news111690272.html
- http://fitsweb.uchc.edu/student/selectives/atolsdorf/Garlic.html
- http://nccam.nih.gov/health/Garlic/ataglance.html
- http://www.ncbi.nlm.nih.gov/pubmed/10515039
- http://sovety-lecheniya.ru/lechebnye-svojstva-chesnoka-recepty-lecheniya.html
- http://natyropat.ru/lekarstvennyie-rasteniya/chesnok-lekarstvennyie-svoystva-retseptyi.html

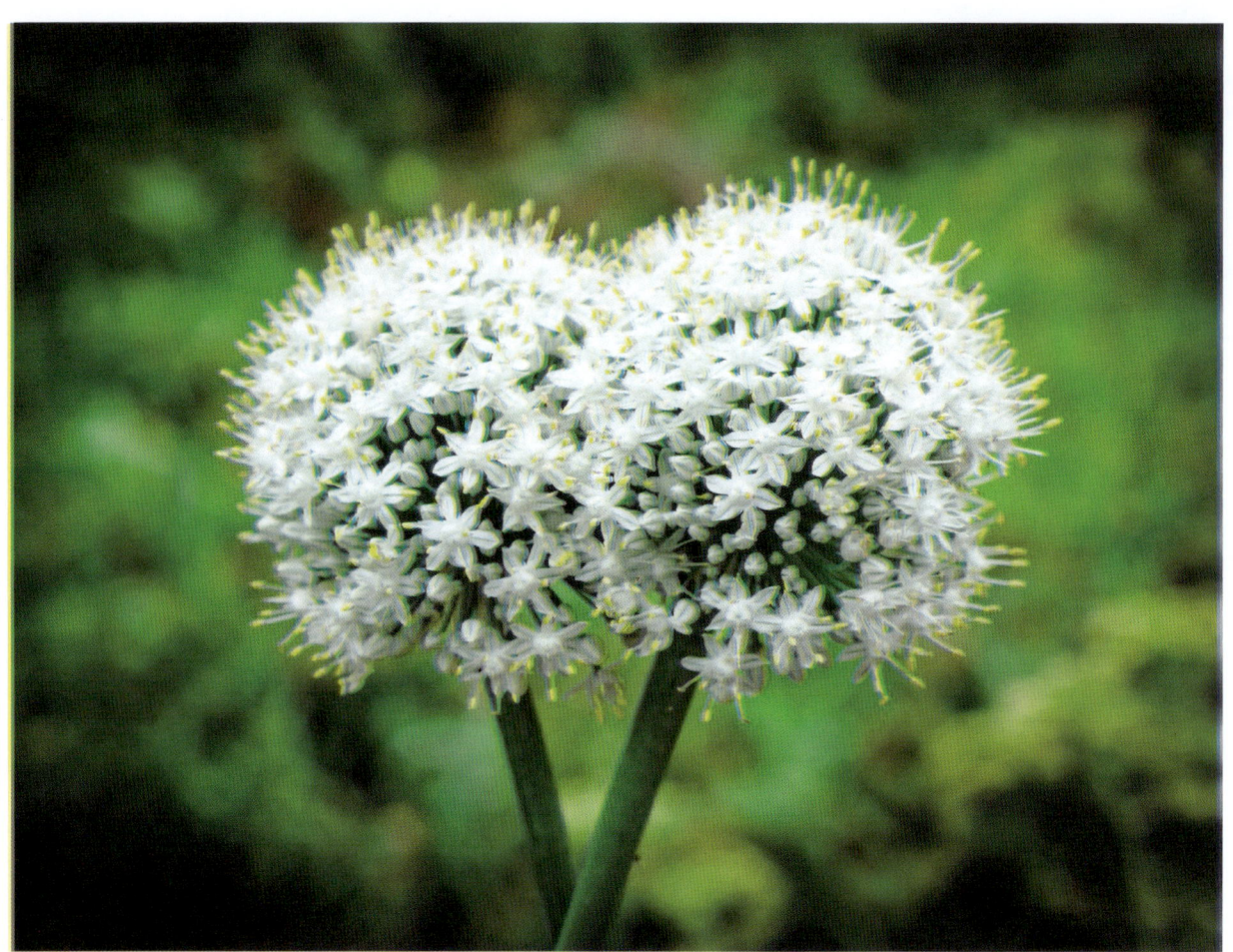

Garlic Flower Essence

Charis Denny

You might be familiar with the images from movies or literature of people trying to repel vampires; villagers cowering behind bolted doors with strings of garlic around their necks, hoping to keep away from Dracula's deadly bite. Or, perhaps you have heard about how effective garlic is for helping your body ward off illness. (If you haven't, you will know all about it after reading this month's issue!) It is one of the best things there is for strengthening your body in its fight against bacteria, germs, and other creepy-crawlies.

Garlic flower essence works in a similar way to ropes of garlic or a tablespoon of fresh garlic honey by shoring up the body's defenses on the physical, emotional, and spiritual levels. It is beneficial to those with low vitality who may be more easily influenced or swayed than others. While garlic flower essence does have an impact on the immune system, it is even better at protecting the user from spiritual or energetic creepy-crawlies. Perhaps most notably, it can prevent the nervous fear that some people experience from not having sufficient protection against foreign energies.

Admittedly, garlic flower essence won't make your spaghetti sauce taste better. But using it does provide you with needed protection and strength for your mind, body, and spirit, as well as guarding you with an active resistance for all parts of your being. And even better, you won't need to chew a mint afterwards!

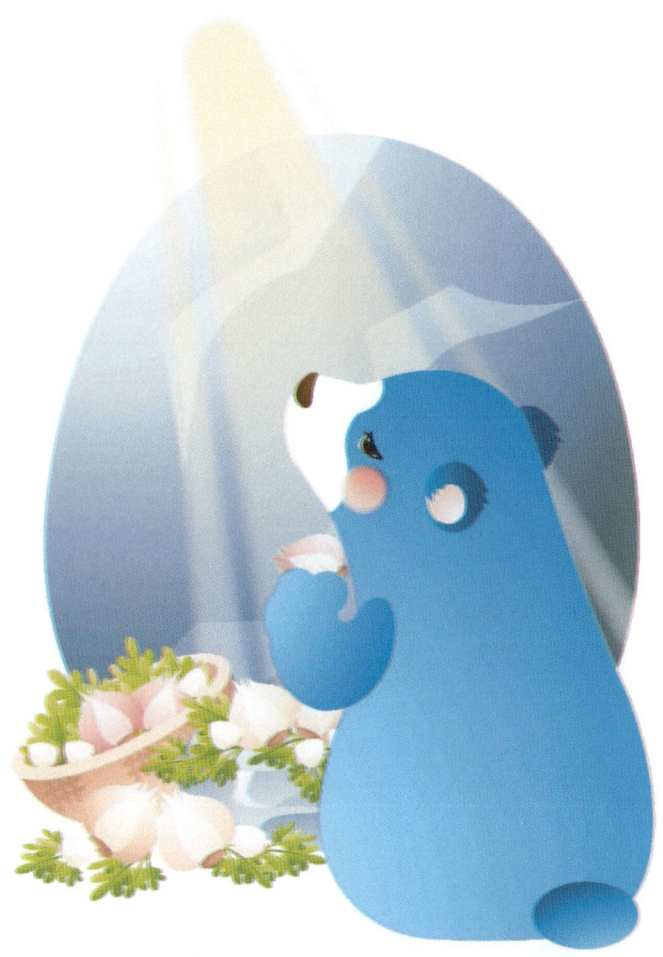

Garlic History and Mythology

Heather Lanham

Garlic, how do I love thee? In so many dishes, and in so many ways. It is my favorite of spices and I use it in nearly every food I eat. I love to pickle it in honey and tamari, though afterward I have to restrain myself from eating an entire jar of garlic. I am not the only lover of garlic; there are so many it is beyond numbers for me. If you were to do an internet search for garlic festivals, you would discover there are pages upon pages of them, and each one in a different locale.

Garlic got its start as a beloved part of so many lives in very early history. Garlic was written about in some of humanities earliest medical texts. Documents from Greece, China, India, Italy, and Egypt all write about medicinal uses for garlic. Cultures that never made contact with each other often found the same uses for garlic. Even modern science is working at confirming many historical uses.

The Egyptians thought garlic as part of the daily food intake was a great way to maintain and increase strength and productivity. It was used for all, be they Kings or Jewish slaves. Garlic was prescribed in Egyptian medical codex as medicine for parasites, insects, circulatory issues, and general malaise.

The Greeks found garlic to be a provider of extra courage, and so fed their military with garlic as part of a daily diet. The Romans felt along the same lines as the Greeks and fed it to their militia as well. Even those who participated in the first Olympic Games ate garlic beforehand in order to enhance performance.

The Ayurvedic medical text, *Charaka Samhita*, mentions garlic as part of a treatment for arthritis and for heart disease. Many ancient medical texts refer to garlic for heart disease and also mention of its use during great plagues. The physics gardens of the Renaissance period often included garlic. Garlic attained such renown that it is even mentioned in the bible. Numbers 11:5 talks of how "We remember the fish which we did eat in Egypt freely; the cucumbers, and the melons, and the leeks, and the onions, and the garlic." Vikings held the humble garlic in high esteem as well, taking healthy supplies of it on every voyage as a fantastic way to aid in health maintenance of the crew on a long journey.

The following are two stories concerning the history of garlic.

Philippines Garlic Legend

"Once upon a time, there live[d] a beautiful maiden. So beautiful that she was sought after by many men. Her mother arranged her wedding with the richest Datus in the village. Each one of them died as her suitors tried hard to impress and win her heart.

The beautiful maiden got sad and was broken hearted about the deaths. She ran to the very top of the sacred mountain where she prayed down on her knees to Bathala. She prayed to take her with him so that her beauty would no longer bring more deaths. Bathala listened to her prayers and call[ed] forth lightning that killed her.

Feeling so much pain, she was buried by her mother where she died. The mother kept on visiting, took good care of the tomb and shed tears.

One day, the mother noticed some grass-like plants growing on her grave. Trying to clean it, the mother pulled them out and realized that the seeds looked like her daughter's teeth. While admiring it, a voice out of nowhere said to her, "those are your daughter's teeth."

In her heart, the mother knew it was Bathala. It is to remind her of her beautiful daughter. The next day, she planted and gave some seeds to her neighbors to spread the memory of her daughter."

Garlic Legend from Korea

"There was once a Heavenly Prince who asked his father, the Heavenly King, to give him the beautiful peninsula of Korea to govern. The King granted his wish and he went down to Korea with three Heavenly seals and 3000 followers. He landed in Korea under a now sacred sandalwood tree. Here he established a sacred city with three ministers to carry out his orders. The ministers were (in English): Earl Wind, Chancellor Rain and Chancellor Cloud. These ministers were in charge of about three hundred and sixty officials who controlled things like grain, life, sickness and the determination of good and evil.

A bear and a tiger who shared a cave near the sacred sandalwood tree wanted very much to become human beings. Every day they prayed so earnestly before the tree that the Heavenly Prince decided to give them a chance to become human. The Heavenly Prince gave the bear and the tiger a bundle of mugwort and twenty bulbs of garlic and told them that if they ate only these and stayed in the cave for one hundred days that they would become human.

So the bear and the tiger took the garlic and the mugwort and went into the cave. After a short time the tiger ran away because it could not stand the long days of sitting [in] the cave and eating only garlic and mugwort, but the bear endured the boredom and the hunger, and after only twenty one days the bear was transformed into a beautiful woman.

The woman was overjoyed, visiting the sandalwood tree again and again she prayed that she may have a child. She became Queen before long and soon gave birth to Dan-Gun the Sandalwood King. Dan-Gun later reigned as the first human King of Korea.

When he became King he moved the capital to [P]yongyang and named the country Zoson (Choson), Land of Morning Calm. Later he moved the capital to Mt. Asadal (Mt. Guwol in Huang-He province) where there is now a shrine called Samsong (the Shrine of the Three Saints) dedicated to the Heavenly King, the Heavenly Prince and Don-Gun. It is said that when Dan-Gun abdicated his throne to the next king that he became a San-sin (Mountain God)."

The Koreans must have considered garlic to be a potent medicine of transformation, to include it here in their creation myth. While I see garlic as transformative, I am happy with it just transforming my food into an even tastier creation.

References
- www.allicinfacts.com/garlic-history
- www.herballegacy.com/Motteshard_History.html
- www.greyduckgarlic.com/The_History_of_Garlic.html
- www.americanfolklore.net/folklore/2010/10/garlic_superstitions_folklore.html
- www.examiner.com/article/myths-and-legends-about-garlic
- www.choosephilippines.com/do/history-and-culture/838/garlic-legend/
- www.natkd.com/korean_creation_myth.http

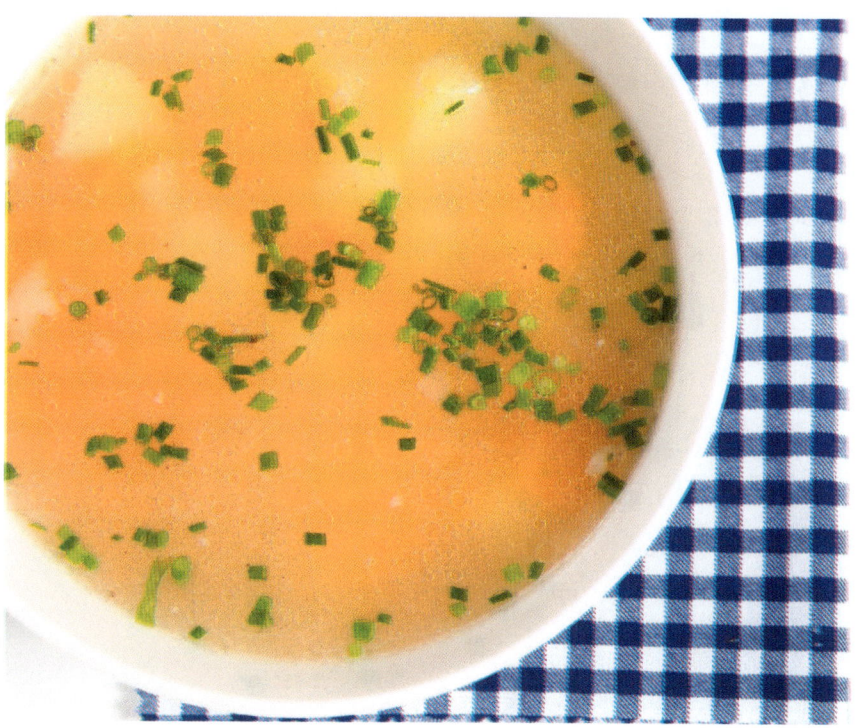

Garlic for Winter Illness

Cassie Soule

Winter illnesses are no fun. The majority of days spent away from work and school over the winter months are due to viral and bacterial illness. There are many herbs out there that can be used to prevent and combat sickness like colds and flu, but none is better than *Allium sativum* – garlic!

Garlic is such an amazing food and herb; it seems that garlic's medicinal benefits can be found whether it is raw, cooked, or taken in capsule form. Most herbalists will say that it is best consumed in the raw form, but studies have shown that chopping garlic and allowing it to sit for 10 minutes before cooking preserves many of the health and medicinal benefits[1]. If you don't like garlic, an easy way to consume it is in capsule form. The benefits found in high quality garlic supplements can be as beneficial as eating it. My go-to brand for garlic supplements is Kyolic. The garlic is aged so the chemical flavor compounds become so mild they are hardly noticeable, yet the medicinal benefits remain.

Garlic is a multifaceted plant that can be used for a variety of health reasons. It can be used daily as a preventative or as an effective medicinal supplement. One of my favorite uses for garlic is for winter illness. These can include cold, flu, ear infections, and respiratory infections of the sinuses and lungs.

The chemical makeup of garlic gives it antibacterial, antiviral, antifungal, anti-inflammatory, and immune boosting actions, which are all commonly known. One of its lesser-known actions is that of an expectorant. These abilities make it extremely appropriate for use in viral and bacterial infections, which include whooping cough (pertussis) and bronchitis.

Not only does *Allium sativum* boost the immune system, but it also supports digestive health, which plays a huge role in immunity. Much of our immune system is found in our gut, so keeping the proper balance of the organisms in the small intestines is very important. Garlic is thought to support beneficial flora while killing harmful bacteria, thus creating an environment for the immune system to work more efficiently.

For ear infections, many herbalists rely on garlic oil for relief. When combined with other herbs like calendula, mullein, chamomile, and lavender, garlic oil has been shown to decrease the duration of the infection due to the antimicrobial and anti-inflammatory benefits of the herbs listed[2].

Garlic is relatively safe for the whole family, especially when consumed in culinary or medicinal amounts. The optimal dose for fresh raw garlic is up to 4 grams daily. It is easy to include it in most meals for prevention purposes, or even in nutritious soups during times of illness. It is also beneficial to a nursing baby when consumed by the mama, and studies suggest that it may increase the frequency of breastfeeding[3]. This is extremely beneficial during times of illness where babies would need to increase their fluids, and much of an infant's immunity is passed on through the breast milk.

We use garlic for medicinal treatment in our home all year long. There is always garlic on my shelf or in the fridge to add to most of the dishes that we eat on a daily basis. Garlic ear oil is a great beginner herbal preparation to make with either the fresh or dried herb. It is a quick yet effective remedy for ear pressure, fullness, and pain. I am blessed with supportive doctors, so I will take my kiddos to have their ears checked when an infection or fluid is suspected. Before committing to any pharmaceutical antibiotic, we use the wait-and-see method along with a few drops of garlic oil applied throughout the day and rarely need the allopathic medicine.

When someone in our family falls to winter illness, one of our favorite food treatments is a warm soup that not only provides great comfort through taste, but also through its medicine. This easy and quick soup can be used as a simple broth if strained or eaten as a hearty meal. Don't worry about the amount of garlic; when boiled it creates a very mild flavor, so add more if you desire. This soup is versatile and can be made to suit your family's tastes and needs.

Garlic Soup

Ingredients

- 16 cloves garlic, peeled and choped
- 1 onion, chopped
- 2 qts of broth
- 2 tsp salt, or to taste
- 6 whole cloves
- 1 tsp dried sage
- 1 tsp dried thyme
- 1 ½ tsp dried oregano
- 3 bay leaves
- 3 Tbsp olive oil

Directions

Simmer all ingredients for 30 minutes. Strain and drink

Optional

Add these ingredients for a healthier meal

- 2 cups of shredded cooked chicken
- 5 chopped carrots
- 3 chopped celery stalks
- 1 cup rice
- ¼ tsp cayenne pepper

Saute veggies and add all optional ingredients to unstrained soup and simmer for the hour. Remove bay leaves and, if possible, remove the spice cloves.

References

1. Heating garlic inhibits its ability to suppress 7, 12-dimethylbenz(a)anthracene-induced DNA adduct formation in rat mammary tissue. Song, K., Milner, JA. March, 1999.

   http://www.ncbi.nlm.nih.gov/pubmed/10082770?dopt=Abstract

2. Naturopathic treatment for ear pain in children. Sarrell EM, Cohen HA, Kahan E. May, 2003.

   http://www.ncbi.nlm.nih.gov/pubmed/12728112

3. Parental influences on Eating Behavior. Savage JS, Fisher JO, Birch LL. 2007

   http://www.ncbi.nlm.nih.gov/pmc/articles/PMC2531152/

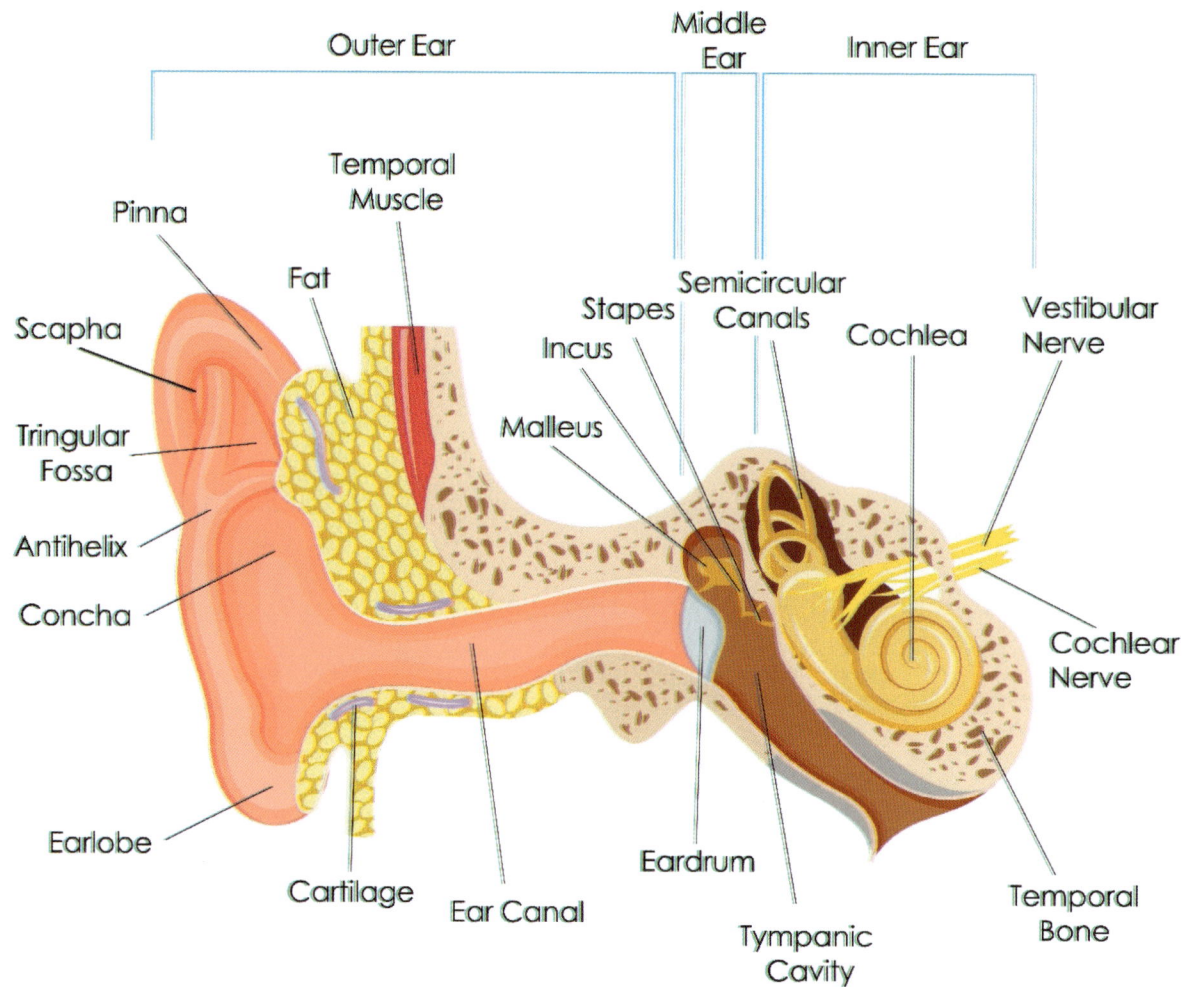

Garlic for Ears

Amanda Klenner

We have and will continue to talk about all sorts of different and delicious ways to incorporate garlic into your life through food. Taking this tasty treatment orally is a great way to get the garlic in, but it isn't the only way to benefit from this great herb.

In many different traditions, from Ayurveda to folk treatment in the hills, garlic has been used to treat infection and inflammation of the ear. We might call this swimmer's ear, or a middle ear infection. Let's talk a bit about the anatomy of the ear before we go much further.

Anatomy

The ear is composed of three general areas. The external consists of the pinna (ear lobe) and external auditory canal where sound enters the ear. The middle ear is where you find the eardrum and the tiny bones behind the ear drum which vibrate – these vibrations are conducted to the cochlea, a part of the inner ear that transforms those vibrations into nerve impulses that are sent to your brain and interpreted as sounds. The inner ear also contains the fluid-filled semicircular canals that are attached to the cochlea and nerves. This inner ear fluid helps your body balance by sending nerve signals to the brain telling it what the head and body position is (standing, sitting, walking, spinning, standing still, etc.). This is why you feel dizzy after spinning in circles – the fluid is still moving even when you have stopped spinning and are standing still. The Eustachian tube is a tube that helps move excess fluid from the inner ears into the throat.

What is an ear infection?

An ear infection is usually defined as pain, redness, or pus in the ear (or leaving the ear) while accompanied by fever. An ear infection can be caused by bacteria or a virus and will usually resolve itself between 48 and 72 hours.

A second type of ear infection called otitis media with effusion (OME), also known as middle ear infection, is an infection that is not usually accompanied by the symptoms listed above, but is diagnosed by fluid buildup behind the ear drum, and is most often the cause of ear tubes.

Ear infections are often caused by viral infections like upper respiratory infections, colds, and flu. Sometimes it is even caused by allergies, either environmental or food. What happens with an OME is fluid builds up in the ears but is unable to drain easily due to inflammation of the area. This can last for a month or more and cause hearing and speech issues in young children. Commonly, doctors will recommend ear tubes for this type of ear infection, especially if it is a chronic or recurring issue. In a review of 41 different studies, researchers found ear tubes did show short shot-term improvement in hearing but found no long-term benefits. These ear tubes also come with some risk, including tympanosclerosis, a calcification of the inner ear that, ironically, can cause hearing loss.

Now, let me interject before I continue, that my husband had chronic hearing issues, dizziness, nausea, and general symptoms of inner ear imbalance. Herbs gave temporary relief but the symptoms kept recurring. When the doctors placed his ear tubes as an adult they found some nasty, viscous gunk in his inner ear that took a while to remove. This was obviously a chronic issue for him and he has seen great improvement from his ear tube placement. What I am saying is weigh your risks, consult with your medical practitioners, and make the best decision you can at the time. There are herbal remedies but sometimes these medical procedures are helpful, so consider your options wisely.

Sometimes antibiotics are effective in the treatment of an ear infection, but they are often overprescribed. Ear infections are the most common reason for a child under the age of 10 to be prescribed antibiotics, but both the American Academy of Pediatrics and the American Academy of Family Physicians have recommended doctors hold off prescribing antibiotics until 48-72 hours after symptoms occur to see if the infection will resolve its self. This is because many ear infections can be caused by viruses, which antibiotics do not treat. They also recommend holding off antibiotic treatment because of the massive outbreak of antibiotic resistant bacteria that we are seeing in our overly sterile world.

What causes ear infections?

Ear infections can happen during or after a viral infection, especially a cold, cough, or any other common disease that affects the upper respiratory system and/or sinuses. They can also happen when water gets trapped in the ears from frequent swimming, food allergies (this is very common for people who have frequent ear infections), seasonal allergies, and spinal misalignment.

How can I treat an ear infection naturally?

The American Academy of Pediatrics recommends waiting 72 hours, but that doesn't mean you have to suffer and hope it resolves on its own. This is the kind of situation where herbal medicine is really allowed to shine. While your doctor may just wait and advice you take Tylenol for the pain, an herbalist will have another solution.

Ear oil is a common, easy, folk treatment to help treat the inflammation, swelling, and infection common to ear infections. Ear oil can be made with many herbs for many different reasons but let me give you two base recipes as well as the herbs I tend to add depending on the person and the symptoms.

Ear Oil Made with Fresh Garlic

This is a remedy you can whip up in your home in minutes and use immediately. If you don't have fresh garlic and oil at your home, you can easily run to the grocery store or your neighbor's house and get some.

Ingredients

- 5-8 garlic cloves, fresh
- ½ C organic oil (olive oil and coconut oil are two of my favorites for this)
- *optional: fresh or dry basil, rosemary, thyme, calendula, mullein flower, or sage

Directions

Crush the garlic and remove the stems. Let the garlic sit and oxidize for 10 minutes. Once that 10 minutes has passed, add your oil to a non-reactive pan and turn the heat to medium/low. Chop your garlic and herbs and add them to the oil.

Sautee on very low, not burning the herbs but slowly frying them and infusing the herbal constituents into the oil. The garlic shouldn't brown, but instead should slightly bubble.

Sautee for 20-30 minutes and allow to cool. NEVER PUT HOT OIL INTO THE EAR.

Once the oil has cooled, place 2-4 drops of the oil into the ear and hold for 5 minutes. Repeat on the other side. Do this 3-4 times a day for 3 days. If symptoms don't resolve, consider following up with your health care provider. If your ear drum has burst, DO NOT PUT ANYTHING IN YOUR EAR. Instead, rub the garlic oil along the sides of your neck where the Eustachian tubes drain into the throat and eat garlic internally to help deal with the infection.

Keep the oil refrigerated and use within 3 days. Throw out after 3 days as botulism can form when you combine fresh herbs (water) and oil.

Are chronic ear infections an issue you often deal with?

First off, look to your diet to see if you have any food sensitivities or allergies that may be causing them. If you have eliminated dietary issues then consider looking to your environment. Are you surrounded by a lot of VOC's off gassing? Artificial fragrance? Dust mites? Mold? There are thousands of things that can cause chronic inflammation. Figure out what is causing your issues and resolve that problem and your ear infections will more than likely become less frequent.

As I mentioned in the previous recipe, the combination of oil and fresh herb with its high water content creates an aerobic environment which is the perfect breeding ground for some nasty bacteria. When an oil goes rancid you can usually tell (the smell is revolting) but one very dangerous bacteria, *Clostridium botulinum* produces the botulism toxin, which can be highly toxic and even fatal at very low doses. Botulism does not cause any identifiable scent or cause a canning lid to bulge. It is a silent toxin. Usually, people over the age of two with healthy digestive and immune systems can handle the botulism toxin internally without death, but why risk it? The botulism toxin is the waste product of the *Clostridium botulinum* organism, which takes about three days to develop. This is why you toss your fresh made oil after three days. You can use it topically with no issues as long as there are no open sores, but do not use a fresh oil internally after three days.

So, when I make product with a long shelf life, I like to make it with fresh dried garlic. This is easy to make. Peel your garlic, slice it thinly and put it onto a dehydrator mat. Dehydrate at 95 degrees until the garlic snaps in half easily. By cutting it and releasing the allicin, then dehydrating it at a low temperature, you are able to retain a lot of the health benefits associated with garlic.

I make up this recipe, put it in ½ oz (15ml) bottles, and dole it out to my friends during swimming season and winter when colds and upper respiratory junk are at their worst. Parts in this case are parts by measurement not by weight so, if you were making this in a 1 quart jar, 1 part would be ½ cup of dried herb.

Dried Garlic Ear Oil

Ingredients

- 1 part dried garlic
- 1 part mullein flower
- 1 part calendula flower, St. John's Wort flower, basil leaf, rosemary leaf, sage leaf, thyme leaf – whatever you have
- organic olive oil

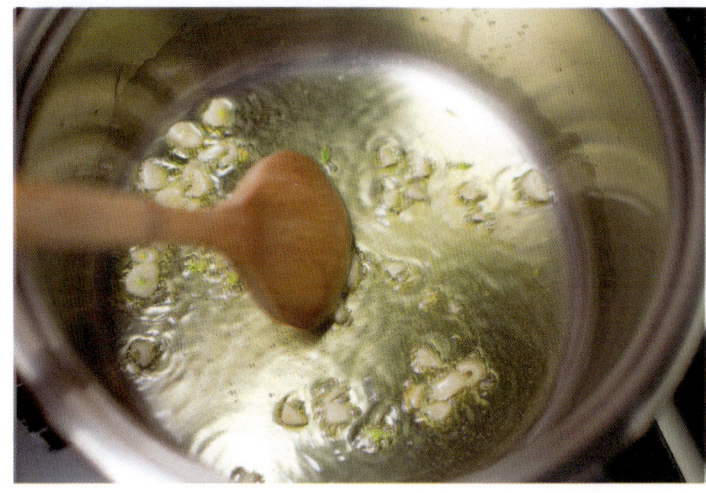

Directions

Place your herbs in a glass mason jar, filling half the jar with dried herb matter. Fill the jar the rest of the way with organic olive oil.

Cap tightly and leave out on a sunny windowsill for 6-8 weeks OR use the double boiler method, and heat the oil in the jar surrounded by water on all sides on low for 12-24 hours.

Strain well, put a tight lid on, and store in a cool dry place. This oil should be used within 1-2 years from the date of production.

Use in the same way as you would the fresh garlic oil.

What do these other herbs do?

Here is a very basic overview of why I include some of these other herbs in my ear oil. Although they are not required, they sure do help.

Mullein flowers are traditionally used for ear infection. In fact, it is most herbalists go-to for ear issues. Mullein flower is anti-inflammatory, analgesic, and is commonly used in animals to treat ear mites. Its leaves do not work as well as the flower, so be sure you are using the right parts! Thankfully, mullein is an invasive weed and can be found in large patches just about anywhere in open sunny spaces.

Calendula is one of my favorite anti-inflammatory, soothing, anti-infective herbs. It does well on most inflamed and irritated membranes internally and externally, making it perfect for ear issues.

St. John's Wort is anti-inflammatory, analgesic, and anti-viral and has been traditionally used to treat ear inflammation, redness, soreness, and pain.

Basil is a personal favorite of mine for ear infection and pain, but the other aromatic herbs (rosemary, sage, thyme etc.) have similar benefits. Aromatic herbs contain a relatively large amount of volatile oils and those listed are specifically anti-bacterial, anti-viral and anti-inflammatory. Although use of the whole herb is generally considered safe, don't put essential oils into your mix. Essential oils are highly concentrated and should not come into contact with your delicate tympanic membrane.

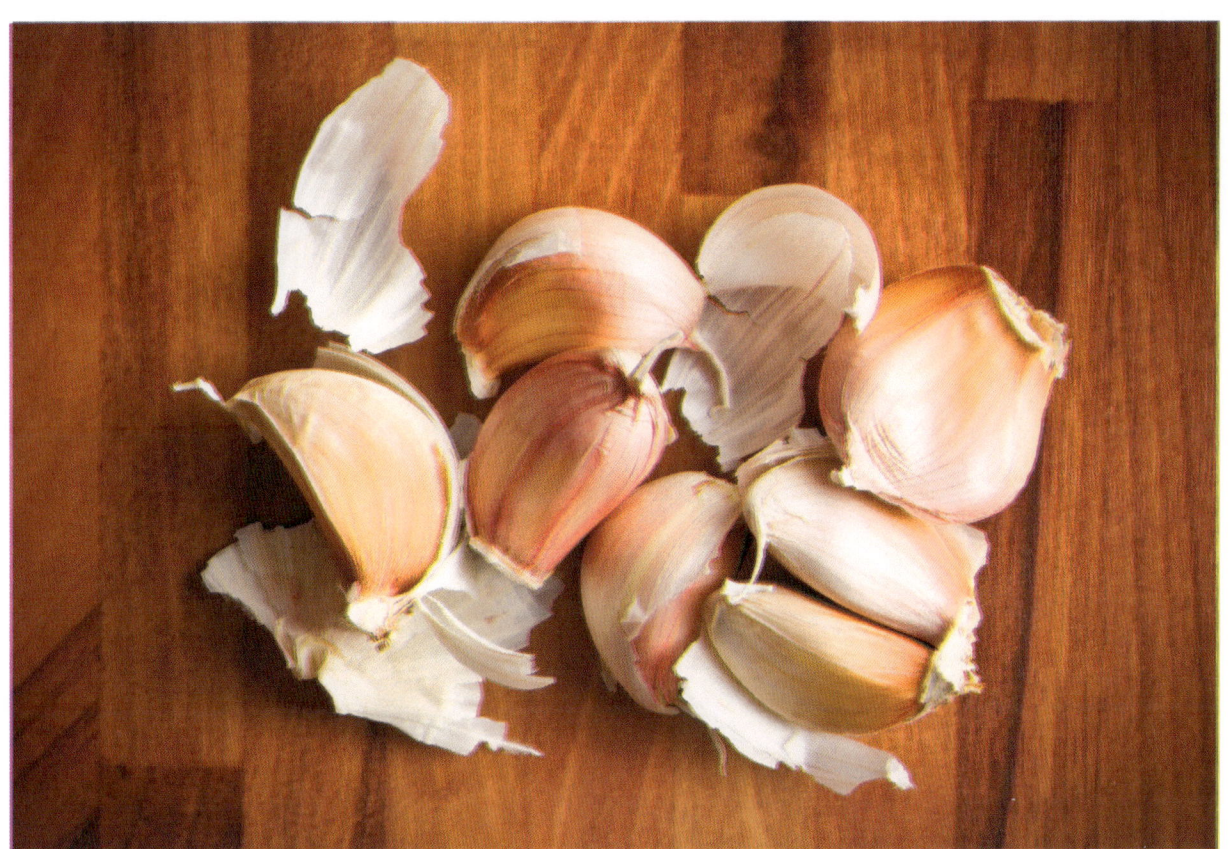

Garlic in the Kitchen: A Powerful Herbal Ally

Carol Little

I absolutely love garlic! Do you? There are so many reasons to include this pungent member of the Amaryllidaceae family in your daily meals, especially now. By incorporating maximum garlic consumption, it offers us so many healing gifts that can really make a huge difference in our own health and our family's well being.

I have even been known to skin garlic cloves and take them as a supplement, just like that; 2 – 3 cloves and a glass of water down the hatch. Most folks, however, would prefer more subtle, shall we say, ways to include this superstar herb into daily meals.

Every year, I visit local farmers' markets and garlic festivals and purchase garlic directly from those who grow it. I enjoy cooking with garlic year round, but have a series of recipes to showcase raw garlic, which has been a part of life in my house for 20+ years.

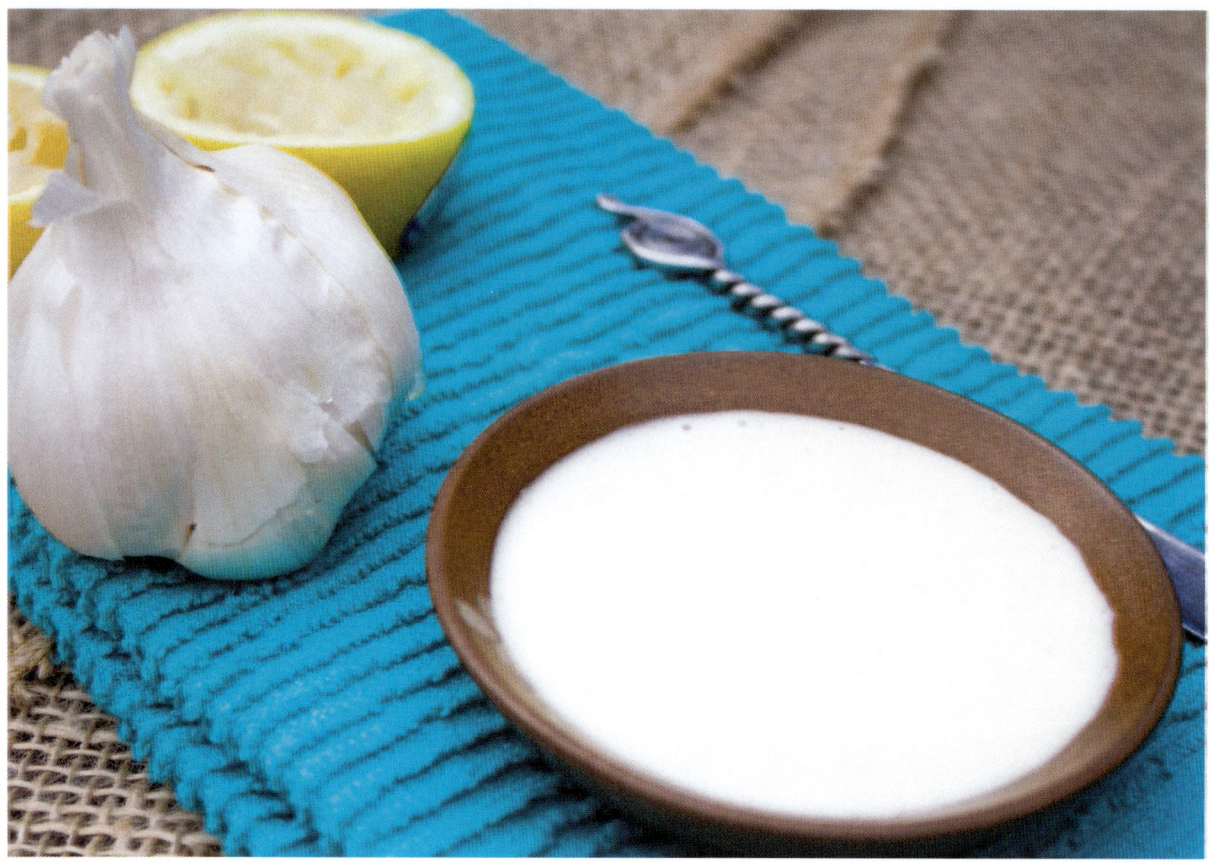

Garlic Paste

Here's a super idea! It is excellent spooned over a baked potato; with any kind of baked chicken, pork, beef, or fish; legumes; and a myriad of vegetables. It takes about 20 minutes to make and stores well in the fridge for 2 weeks (or freezes well). *Vampires beware!*

Ingredients

- 2 bulbs garlic, cloves separated and peeled (8-12 cloves)
- ½ C lemon juice (freshly squeezed if possible)
- ¾ tsp sea salt
- 1 – 1 ½ C good quality extra virgin olive oil
- 1 egg white (optional)

Directions

Put all of the garlic and the egg white (if using) in a blender or food processor and blend until garlic is chopped. Add ¼ cup of the lemon juice and the salt. Pulse until combined.

Slowly add a small amount, about ¼ cup, of the oil. Blend until the mixture becomes slightly smooth, at least one minute. Add another ¼ cup oil and continue to blend. Add the remaining lemon juice and blend for another minute.

Continue to add oil and blend for about a minute until 1 cup of oil has been added. We are looking for a smooth, thick, garlicky paste. If the garlic bulbs are large, the recipe may require additional oil. Stop adding oil when the oil itself stops blending into the mixture.

The mixture should become thick and resemble golden mayonnaise.

Pickled Garlic

It's been 20 years since my dear friend and mentor Rosemary Gladstar taught me how to pickle garlic three ways. I honestly can't tell you which I prefer, because I enjoy each, but will include all here. Make them both and YOU decide!

They will be either salty-sweet or tart-sweet. The degree of sweetness can also be adjusted, so as with many adventures with herbs, the recipes are more of a guide than a recipe. Use your imagination!

Ingredients

- garlic bulbs, amount will vary
- tamari OR apple cider vinegar OR both
- honey
- glass jar (I tend to use a canning jar)

Directions

Peel several heads of garlic. Try not to nick the cloves, as this will make them turn black or brown. (This doesn't affect the result or the taste, but cloves in their original color look more appetizing.) Place the cloves in a glass jar. Choose the size of jar carefully; the idea is to have the garlic cloves piled in the jar and topped with liquid so that there's not a lot of air space.

Cover the garlic cloves with tamari or apple cider vinegar* and allow to steep in a warm area (ideally a warm cupboard) for 4-8 weeks. Sometimes air bubbles will form, but this is a part of the process. Ensure that the cloves are always covered with liquid.

After 4 – 8 weeks, strain the liquid into a bowl or another jar. Pour ½ to 1 cup of the liquid into a measuring cup. Add an equal amount of honey. Mix together and pour the sweetened mixture back into the original jar, over the garlic cloves.

The remaining unused portion of the liquid makes a delicious addition to sauces, stews, and salad dressings.
Put a tight-fitting lid onto the jar with the garlic and allow to sit another 4 -8 weeks.

The result yields a tasty, raw garlic condiment with all of the power of garlic's goodness. It can be taken daily as a preventative or used with salads or many main dish meals.

*Use tamari, apple cider vinegar, or both! If time permits, I like to make all three. If not? I make the version with both tamari and apple cider vinegar. Tamari is a fermented Japanese version of the common soy sauce. It offers a deeper, richer flavor and is available gluten free.

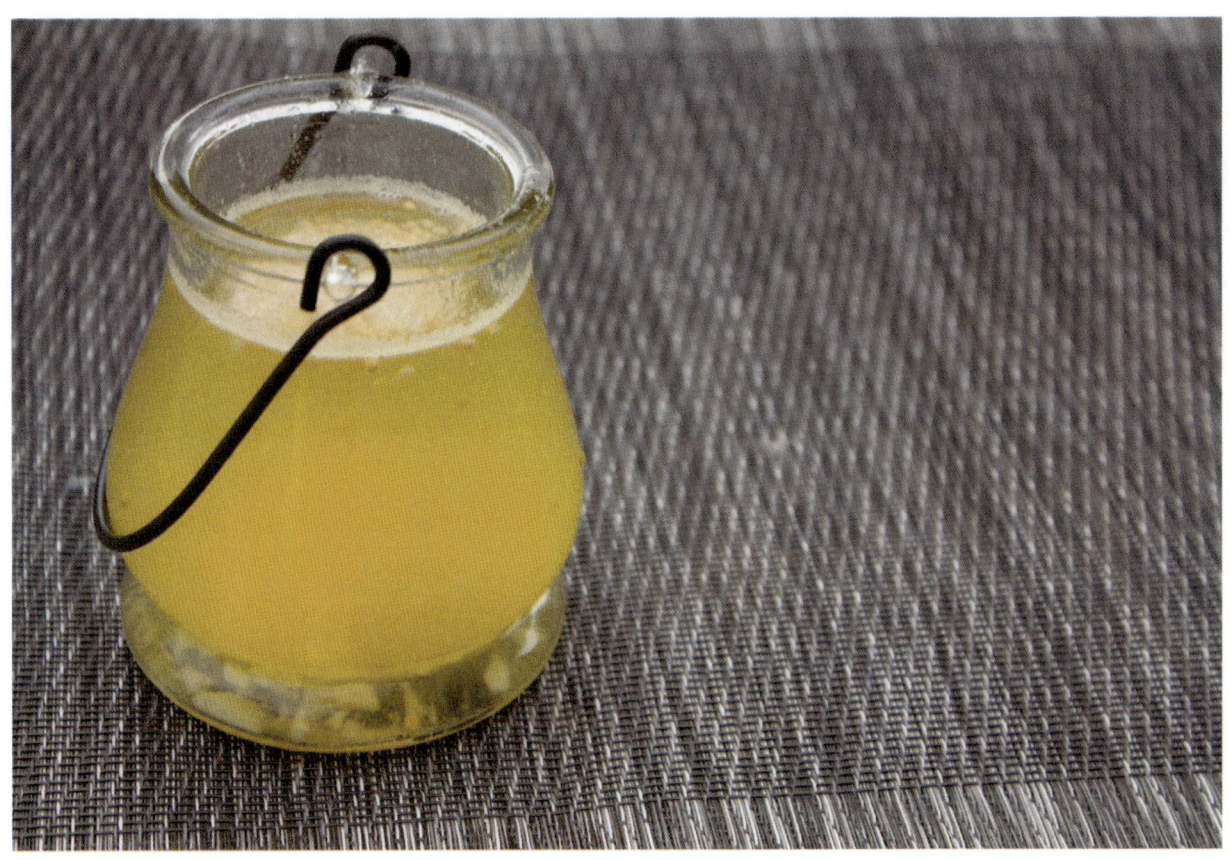

Garlic Syrup

Looking for a way to take in the best of garlic as a homemade supplement or easy to administer healing syrup? It's easy to make.

Ingredients

- 2 C pure water
- 1 ½ C fresh garlic, chopped
- 1 Tbsp fennel seeds
- 1 tsp cumin seeds
- 1 tsp coriander seeds
- 1 C raw honey, local if possible
- apple cider vinegar (optional)
- stainless steel, glass, or other non-reactive pot

Directions

Add the garlic and water to a pot and add the seeds. Boil until garlic is soft. Transfer to a glass jar with a lid and allow to steep for 8-12 hours.

Put the mixture back into the pot andadd the cup of honey (or a bit more if necessary) to make a syrup consistency. If using, add a little apple cider vinegar and bring to a boil. Remove from the heat and allow to cool. Store in a glass jar. I find that canning jars are invaluable in general, and I use one for this recipe as well.

Take a teaspoon every morning or more often if in acute stage of cold/flu/congestion. I like this combination of herbs but you can make adjustments to include your personal favorites.

Garlic Syrup- Quick Version

No time to make the above concoction but want a quick remedy? Here's an idea:

Ingredients

- several bulbs of garlic
- raw honey
- glass canning jar

Directions

Slice several bulbs of garlic and put into a clean canning jar. Add raw honey to cover the garlic. Place tight-fitting lid on the jar and set aside.

In the next 48 hours, the juice from the garlic will mix with the honey. Take 1-2 teaspoons of this syrup every 30 minutes for congestion in the lungs and to relieve cough spasms or a sore throat.

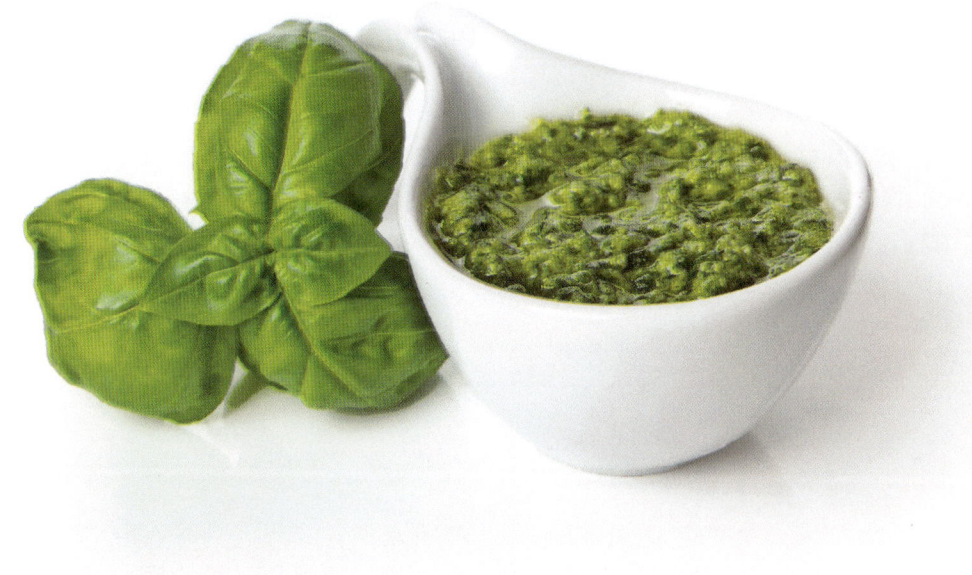

Garlic Scapes Pesto

This is one of my all-time favorite pesto recipes! Garlic scapes impart a mild garlic flavor and can be enjoyed cooked or raw. Chop them into a salad or use in recipes calling for green onions or scallions. They are delicious when sautéed with mushrooms, celery, peppers, or your favorite veggies in a quick stir-fry, and then pair extremely well atop whole grain or rice pasta, even served over a dish of spelt, quinoa, or other whole grain.

Ingredients

- 1 C grated Parmesan cheese (or Romano)
- 3 Tbsp fresh lime or lemon juice
- ¼ lb garlic scapes (110g)
- ½ C olive oil

Directions

Puree garlic scapes and olive oil in a food processor until smooth. Remove from processor and stir in Parmesan and lime juice. Add seasoning to taste.

Serve on bread, crackers, pasta, or as a dip for raw or grilled veggies. I always make extra and freeze it in ice cube trays overnight. Afterwards, I pop them into labeled freezer bags for easy access and a delicious + nutritious garlicky "pop" to many meals. They thaw easily and can be a super quick pasta sauce, tossed with BBQ veggies, or stirred into your favorite grain dish. It has limitless possibilities!

This is one of my all-time preferred quick recipes to make when feeling a bit under the weather. We can't go wrong with a combination of healing constituents from these plant medicines!

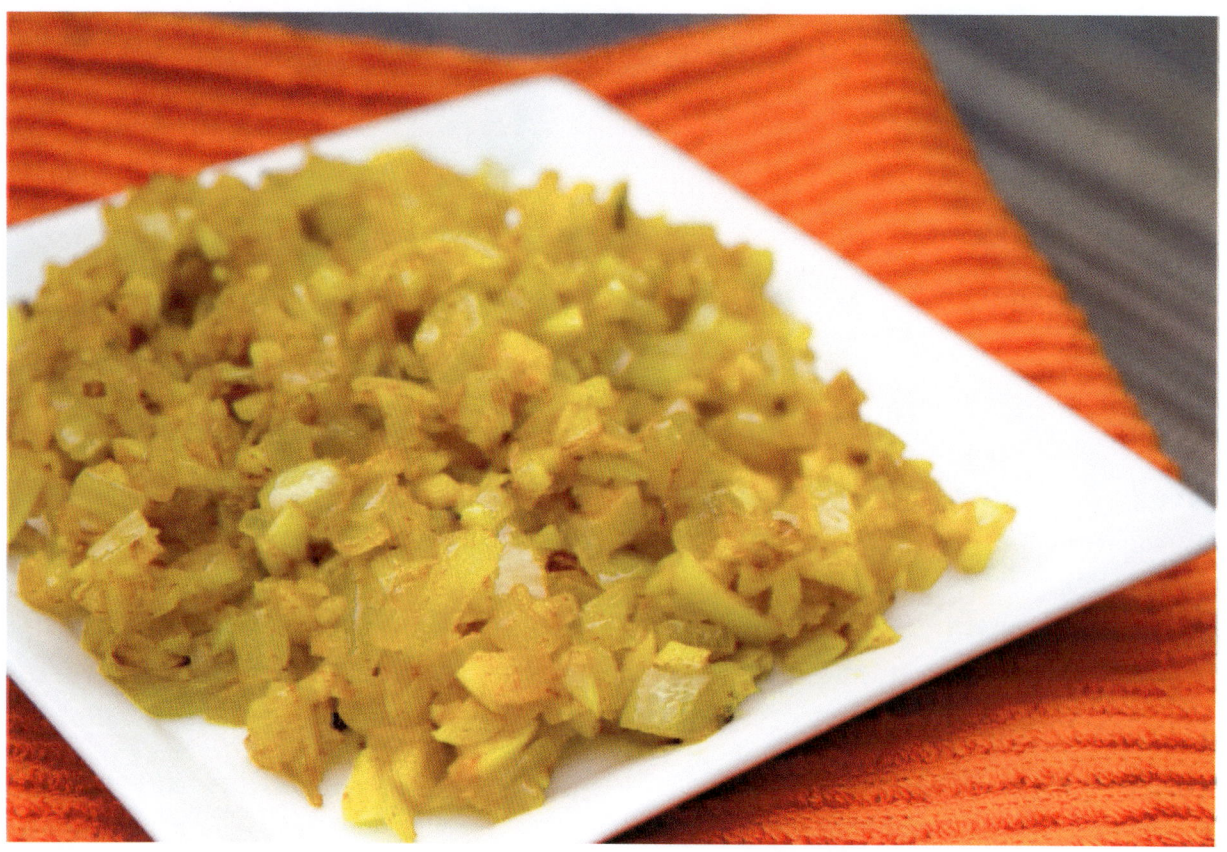

Garlic, Onions & Curry Sauté

The curry powder can be substituted with another herb or herbal blend that you find delicious. I've made this with garlic, onions and Italian spice blends, for example, with great results. However, the turmeric in the mild curry powder that I use offers additional healing components.

Ingredients

- 1 garlic bulb, cloves split, peeled, and chopped
- 1-2 medium onions, sliced
- 1-2 tsp curry (or turmeric or herbal blend of your choice)
- 1-2 cracks of black pepper
- olive or coconut oil

Directions

Slice onions and sauté in a small amount of olive oil or coconut oil. Add ½ of the garlic to the onions when they are translucent. Toss lightly and stir frequently to avoid burning the garlic. Add the curry powder (or your preference) and stir. Add the remaining garlic. Allow the garlic to heat through and remove the pan from heat.

This concoction is best eaten warm. The onions are sweet, garlic pungent, and the curry flavorful.

Whichever way you choose to enjoy glorious garlic, I hope you have fun experimenting with some of these ideas and find your own favorites. Garlic is good!

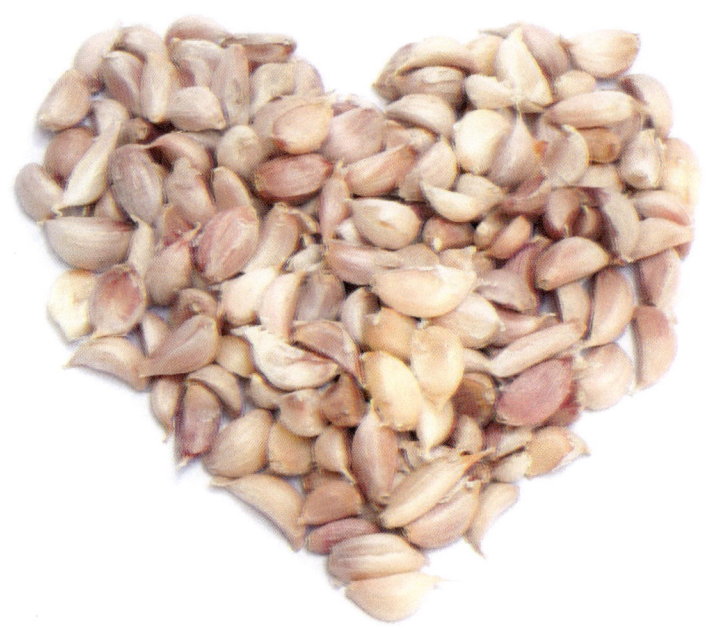

Heart Healthy Garlic

Angela Justis

Among its many uses, garlic is a wonderful herbal ally for protecting and restoring health to the cardiovascular system. Wisdom gained from traditional usage combined with modern research shows us the benefits of garlic for the heart. Garlic's healing properties address many of the factors that contribute to cardiovascular disease including, atherosclerosis and hypertension. Because cardiovascular disease is rampant in the world today, garlic is an important herb for prevention and healing of these unfortunately common problems.

Hardening of the arteries, or atherosclerosis, is a major contributor to cardiovascular disease. It happens when deposits composed of fat, cholesterol, and other substances are made along arterial walls. Over time blockages form, impeding blood flow and ultimately causing decreased circulation to organs. This can even lead to a heart attack or stroke. Garlic offers wonderfully rich antioxidant sulfur containing compounds that help to protect blood vessels from inflammation and damaging oxidation. Damage to the vessels and cells of the circulatory system through oxidation and inflammation increases the risk of plaque formation and subsequent blockages. Garlic also works to lower serum LDL (bad cholesterol) and triglycerides while increasing HDL (good cholesterol) and inhibiting platelet aggregation along blood vessel walls. It may also help to remove any existing deposits, helping folks suffering from atherosclerosis.

Hypertension, or high blood pressure, is another major contributor to cardiovascular disease. Trusty garlic is a hypotensive that helps to regulate arterial tension. Regular consumption taken over a period of time will help to lower high blood pressure.

Heating, stimulating, and drying, garlic encourages and improves circulation. It's vasodilating effect opens up the arteries and improves circulation to the whole body, including the periphery. Furthermore, garlic is an anticoagulant and antithrombotic that helps keep the blood flowing smoothly while preventing blood clot formation. These actions help ensure healthy blood flow and the prevention of both heart attacks and strokes.

Garlic is easy to use! Simply adding it to your diet is a wonderful way to benefit from its many virtues. Dosages for supplementation of garlic for heart health are wide and varied. Most herbalists agree that garlic is best taken raw and freshly chopped or pressed. This is because one of the most helpful components of garlic is a substance called allicin that forms during an enzymatic reaction that occurs when garlic is crushed or chopped. Allicin degrades very quickly with time and upon exposure to heat, so garlic is best consumed raw. Take 1 to 3 small cloves of crushed garlic or 15 to 40 drops of tincture made from fresh garlic, not dried, 3 times per day.

Consumption of fresh, raw garlic will likely give you bad breath and may irritate your stomach. Take garlic with food to decrease stomach irritation and eat something with chlorophyll, such as mint or parsley, to combat garlic breath. Studies conducted with aged garlic extract and powdered garlic have found these preparations to be viable forms of supplementation. For these, follow package directions.

Take the wisdom of the ancients and the research of modern day scientists to heart! Know that not only is garlic a tasty addition to your diet, it is a wonderful choice for keeping your cardiovascular system healthy and strong.

A Special Note on Safety: If you have a heart condition, please be sure to work closely with your doctor when taking herbs, especially if you are on medication, as herbs can easily have unexpected reactions with prescription drugs.

References

Books

- Gladstar, Rosemary, *Family Herbal*, Storey Books, 2001
- Green, James, *The Male Herbal*, The Crossing Press, 1991
- Hoffman, David, *The Complete Illustrated Herbal*, Element Books, 1996
- Kutts & Chereau, *Naturae Medicina*, Rocky Mountain Herbalists Coalition, 1990
- McIntyre, Anne, *Flower Power*, Henry Holt & Company, Inc., 1996
- Tilgner, Sharol, N.D., *Herbal Medicine from the Heart of the Earth*, Wise Acres Press, Inc., 1999

Websites

- http://jn.nutrition.org/content/136/3/736S.long
- http://www.nutritionj.com/content/1/1/4
- http://www.hindawi.com/journals/ecam/2013/125649
- http://www.ncbi.nlm.nih.gov/pubmed/16484553
- http://www.heartmdinstitute.com/nutrition/healthy-diet/76-dr-sinatras-top-healing-spices
- http://circ.ahajournals.org/content/99/4/591.full
- http://articles.mercola.com/sites/articles/archive/2013/09/23/garlic-health-benefits.aspx
- http://www.whfoods.com/genpage.php?tname=foodspice&dbid=60

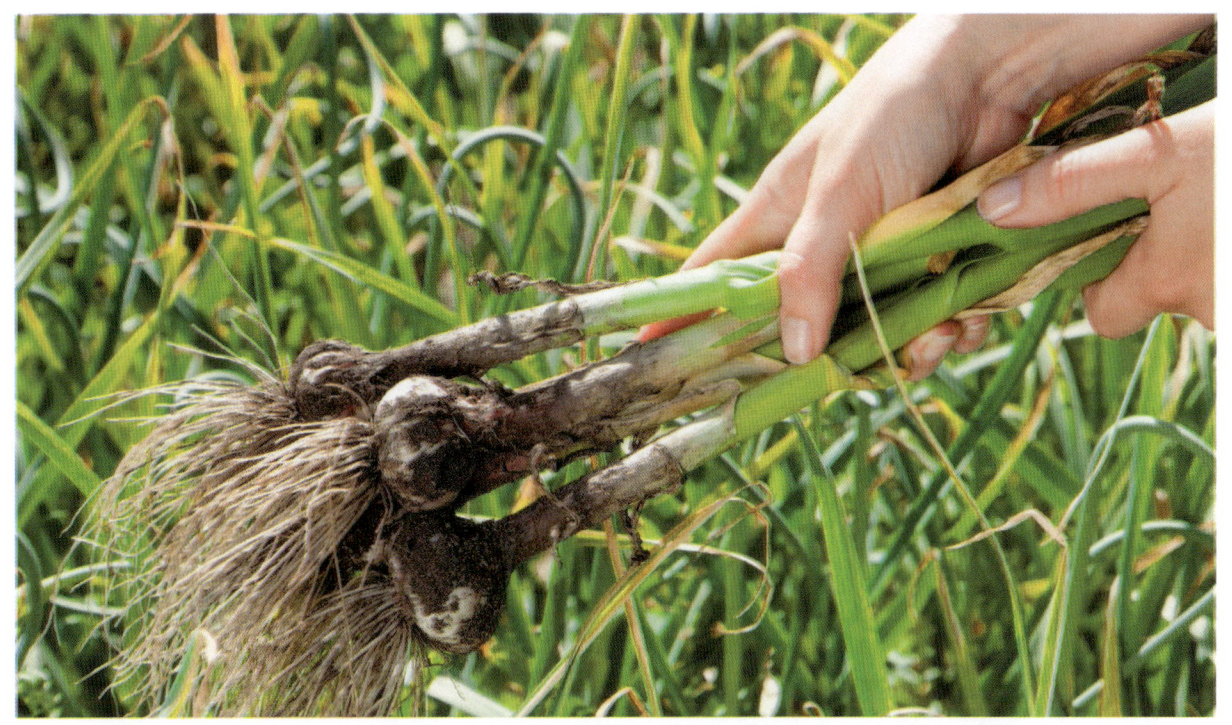

Garlic is as Good as Ten Mothers!

Jessica Morgan

I once heard that dreaming about "garlic in the house" brings good luck and the discovery of hidden secrets. I'm really not surprised, are you? There are so many objects and symbols that are said to bring good luck and fortune, but I think the one thing that holds garlic above and beyond all those other symbols of good fortune is immune strength and good health! Plus, it's yummy, delicious, and as good as ten mothers! But passed down in legend, fairy tales, and numerous superstitions throughout history, on every continent, and within every culture on earth, there is a link in the story of garlic. The one link that ties them all together is that garlic has the power to protect from harm and diseases, can ward off the evil spirits, and brings good luck. I call that a good luck charm worth keeping around. Don't you?

Garlic is cheap and readily available at the grocery store, but people who like to grow their own herbs and veggies might enjoy harvesting garlic from their own gardens too. Being an effective control for many pests makes it a huge value to both the organic garden and the organic gardener. There's no secret that it's easy to grow, easy to cook, and easy to make medicine with. And now's the time to plant!

Common Name Garlic, ajo, allium, stinking rose, rustic treacle, nectar of the gods, camphor of the poor, and poor man's treacle.

Botanical Name *Allium sativum.* The name comes from *allium*, a Celtic word meaning burning or smarting, and *sativum* meaning cultivated.

Best Climate and Site Zones 7-10, ideally in full sun.

Ideal Soil Condition Rich, well-drained soil: pH 4.5-8.3.

Growing Guidelines Garlic is one of the easiest of all vegetables to grow, provided you have a suitable sunny site. Propagate from cloves. Garlic needs a cold period to trigger growth, so your cloves should be planted in the late fall. Plant the cloves with the pointed side up. Do not separate cloves from the bulb until just before you are ready to plant them, or they may dry out. Plant 6 inches apart and 2 inches deep. Prepare as for onions; dig well, loose ground. For largest bulbs, prune away flowering stems that shoot up in early summer. In severe-winter areas, plant in early spring.

Growing Habit Perennial bulb: height up to two feet. Depending on variety, foliage resembles onions, iris, or tulips.

Flowering Time Early summer; small, white to pinkish blooms flower atop a tall central stem.

Pests and Disease Prevention Avoid over-watering the soil to prevent bulb disease, but garlic is generally trouble free. Beyond its intense flavor and culinary uses, "the stinking rose" is good in the garden as an insect repellent. It's known to protect against borers when grown around fruit trees, and is also considered an effective destroyer of the diseases that damage stone fruits, cucumbers, radishes, spinach, brand, nuts, and tomatoes. And furthermore, an experiment conducted at the University of California showed when a garlic-based oil was sprayed on breeding pods, there was a 100 percent kill of mosquito larvae.

Harvesting and Storing Dig bulbs after tops begin to fall over, and before bulb skins begin to decay underground. Place them in a single layer in a shady spot to dry, then cut away tops or braid together.

Parts Used Bulbs, scapes

Culinary Uses Adds flavor to most meats, seafood, and vegetables. Raw garlic is used in sauces and added as a condiment to butter, vinegar, and salt.

Lore The history of the alliums go way back way before recorded time, but one Egyptian record mentions the roundness of onions, thought by priests, was a symbol of the whole universe. The onion layers, one on top of the other, seemed to copy the layers of heaven, earth, and hell. And, in fact, an old Turkish legend says the strong odor of onion dates back to when Satan was thrown out of heaven and onions grew where he put his right foot, smelly garlic where he put his left.

Garlic as a Companion Plant Plant garlic with tomatoes and roses.

Recipes

"One must be suspicious of anyone who does not eat garlic" – Ancient Roman proverb

I think that garlic should not only be eaten daily, but also incorporated into our daily tonics and foods. Here are a few of my favorite ways to use my homegrown garlic – in vinegar, because if garlic is as good as ten mothers, then in vinegar it must be as good as twenty!

Traditional Fire Cider

Fire Cider is an old-fashioned, vinegar-based herbal tincture often made with fresh onions, garlic, horseradish, ginger, and cayenne, although the formula can be varied any way you like it. It has superior immune stimulant properties: is antimicrobial, antiviral, antibacterial, and anti- fungal. In addition, fire cider has diaphoretic and vasodilating properties. It increases the blood flow and the amount of oxygen delivered to the tissues, as well as aids in the removal of waste products from the tissues. All of the herbs contained inside have expectorant properties, making it valuable for the first phases of a cold or flu or for lowered resistance. It is an adjunct treatment for sinusitis, bronchitis, allergies, poor circulation, and for digestive infections.

Ingredients

- raw apple cider vinegar, such as Braggs
- 4-inch piece chopped ginger rhizome
- 4-inch piece chopped horseradish root
- 1 small chopped onion
- 1 bulb chopped garlic
- 2-3 cayenne peppers or 1 Tbsp powdered cayenne*
- honey to taste

*You can use any kind of fresh or dried hot peppers ranging from mild to hot. I prefer cayenne powder 90,00 H.U. Other options that enhance both the flavor and nutritional value are as follows: include herbs such as elderberries, turmeric, burdock, basil, oregano, or thyme – be creative! I sometimes add seaweed to the recipe to increase the vitamin and nutrient content like I do in my bone broths. Just don't forget to write your recipes down. Also, feel free to leave out the cayenne or the horseradish if you have a hot constitution. Add marshmallow root or lemons instead! Anything goes in your cider.

Directions

Peel the skin off both the onions and garlic. Chop onions, garlic, and peppers – be careful not to touch your eyes! The horseradish and ginger can be grated or finely chopped.

Place the ingredients into a sterilized mason jar, filling the jar one to two inches below the mouth. Pour the vinegar over the herbs, making sure there are no air bubbles. Cap with a plastic lid. Allow the herbs to steep for 3-4 weeks in a dark place, then strain off the liquid and bottle.

To Use: Take 1-4 droppers full, 3-5 times daily or as a tonic. You can also use Fire Cider in place of vinegar in your recipes.

Four Thieves Vinegar

This vinegar is said to have been used to prevent catching the Black Death during the medieval period. Other similar types of herbal vinegars have been used as medicine since the time of Hippocrates, and adding antiviral, antibacterial, and antifungal herbs to your vinegar makes for really potent medicines that are useful for the common cold and flu, or as a tonic for everyday immune health. Each herb represents one of the thieves so traditionally there were four herbs in the vinegar, but I like to make it a little more powerful with a few garlic cloves

Ingredients

- raw apple cider vinegar, such as Braggs
- 2 cloves smashed garlic
- 2 Tbsp fresh thyme
- 2 Tbsp fresh sage
- 2 Tbsp fresh lavender
- 2 Tbsp fresh mint

Directions

Place 2 crushed garlic cloves in a jar and then layer the herbs over them. Pour the vinegar over the herbs and seal tightly with a plastic lid (metal lids will corrode). Leave it in a cool, dark place for 3-4 weeks, shaking every few days if possible. Strain off the liquid and bottle. To Use: Take 1-4 droppers full, 3-5 times daily when feeling ill or as a tonic.

Be creative! You can add all kinds of different herbs if you want, like rosemary!

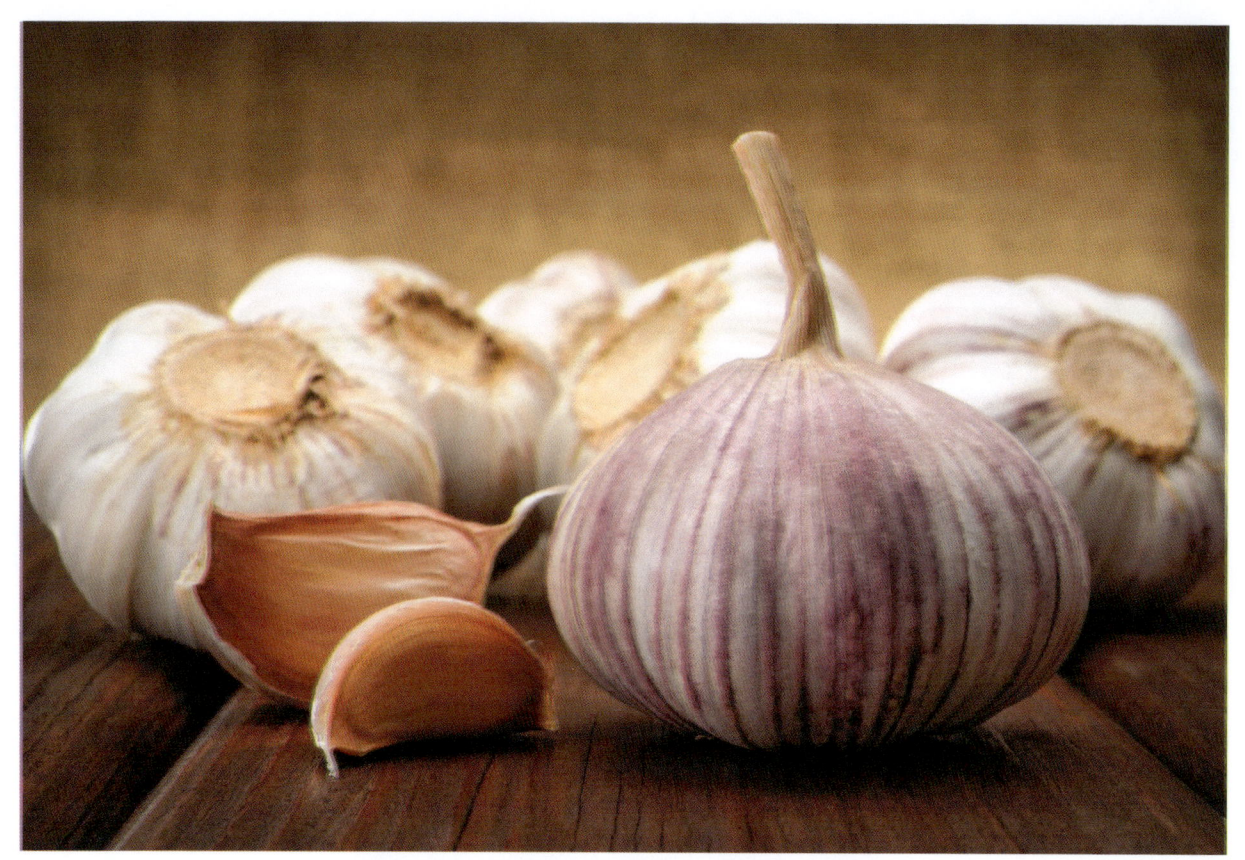

Get the Garlic In

Marlene Adelmann

There are very sound reasons to "get the garlic in" when we are planning immune boosting meals or addressing the sudden onset of colds and flu. Garlic can be eaten as a food and can be a delicious addition to kid-friendly recipes. It is useful chopped up and used in syrups made with honey or maple syrup with a little lemon added. It can also be used externally on the skin as a transdermal application.

Garlic is a great source of vitamin C, and it also contains vitamins B-6 and B-1, manganese, potassium, selenium, calcium, and iron. Garlic helps us fight infection with its antibacterial and antiviral properties found in the compound allicin. If taken immediately and at regular intervals, it offers a quick arsenal against the first signs of cold or flu infection.

Infections occur when bacteria, viruses, and other pathogens enter the body and begin to multiply. It is best to treat symptoms early on to help arrest the multiplying action of the infection, thereby lessening the duration and effect on the body.

The healing properties in the allicin are most present in the raw garlic clove and are greatly diminished by cooking, so we have to do a little planning here to get our little ones to eat raw, stinky garlic or take it in its raw form as a remedy.

From the Outside In

Make a garlic patch using a piece of cheesecloth or paper towel, a bit of olive oil, and some crushed garlic cloves.

Note: topical applications of garlic can be caustic and have been known to cause chemical burns on the skin of both children and adults. Always conduct a patch test first and monitor the patch continuously for adverse effects. If a reaction occurs, discontinue use.

Cut and fold over a few pieces of cheesecloth or paper towel. Pour a drop or two of olive oil onto the cloth and then add 3-4 crushed garlic cloves, and place this patch on or near the part of the body that you are treating. For colds and flu, a patch can be placed on the chest or throat area. Leave in place for 5-10 minutes. Repeat every hour using fresh crushed garlic.

Goot

Ingredients

- 10-12 garlic cloves, chopped
- 4 Tbsp coconut oil
- 4 Tbsp olive oil
-

Directions

Make goot by placing 4 tablespoons of coconut oil in a saucepan; heat over low heat until melted. Remove the pan from the stove and add 4 tablespoons of olive oil along with 10-12 chopped raw garlic cloves. Place this mixture in a blender and blend for 2 minutes. Remove any large pieces of garlic by pouring the mixture through a sieve. Goot can be kept in a glass jar in the refrigerator for up to two weeks. The paste can be applied directly to the skin for absorption, carrying with it all the beneficial properties for fighting infections. Goot can be applied to the soles of children's feet where the skin is less sensitive, and further away from the nose! Again, because topical garlic has been associated with burns in children, be sure to conduct a small patch test first.

We have all known children that we refer to as "good eaters." They enjoy an extensive repertoire of good foods from kale soup to raw, delicious nuts! Then there are the "fussy eaters" who seem to exist on PB and J sandwiches and mac and cheese. We look at these kids askance and wonder how is it that they continue to thrive on such meager nutrition. Well, somehow they do, and many of them will begin to enjoy a more balanced diet that includes healthier foods as they grow. All the while these "good eaters" are tossing back spinach, tomatoes, and juicy cucumbers. We are probably going to have an easier time getting the garlic into the good eaters, but what about the fussbudgets? Here are some thoughts and recipes to consider:

To get the most benefit from garlic, it should be eaten raw. A good idea is to chop up fresh garlic and add it to any recipe at the end of the cooking process. Add chopped or crushed raw garlic to spaghetti sauce, soups, egg dishes, pizza, flat breads, and pasta dishes. Try garlic butters, garlicky mashed potatoes, and creamy cauliflower.

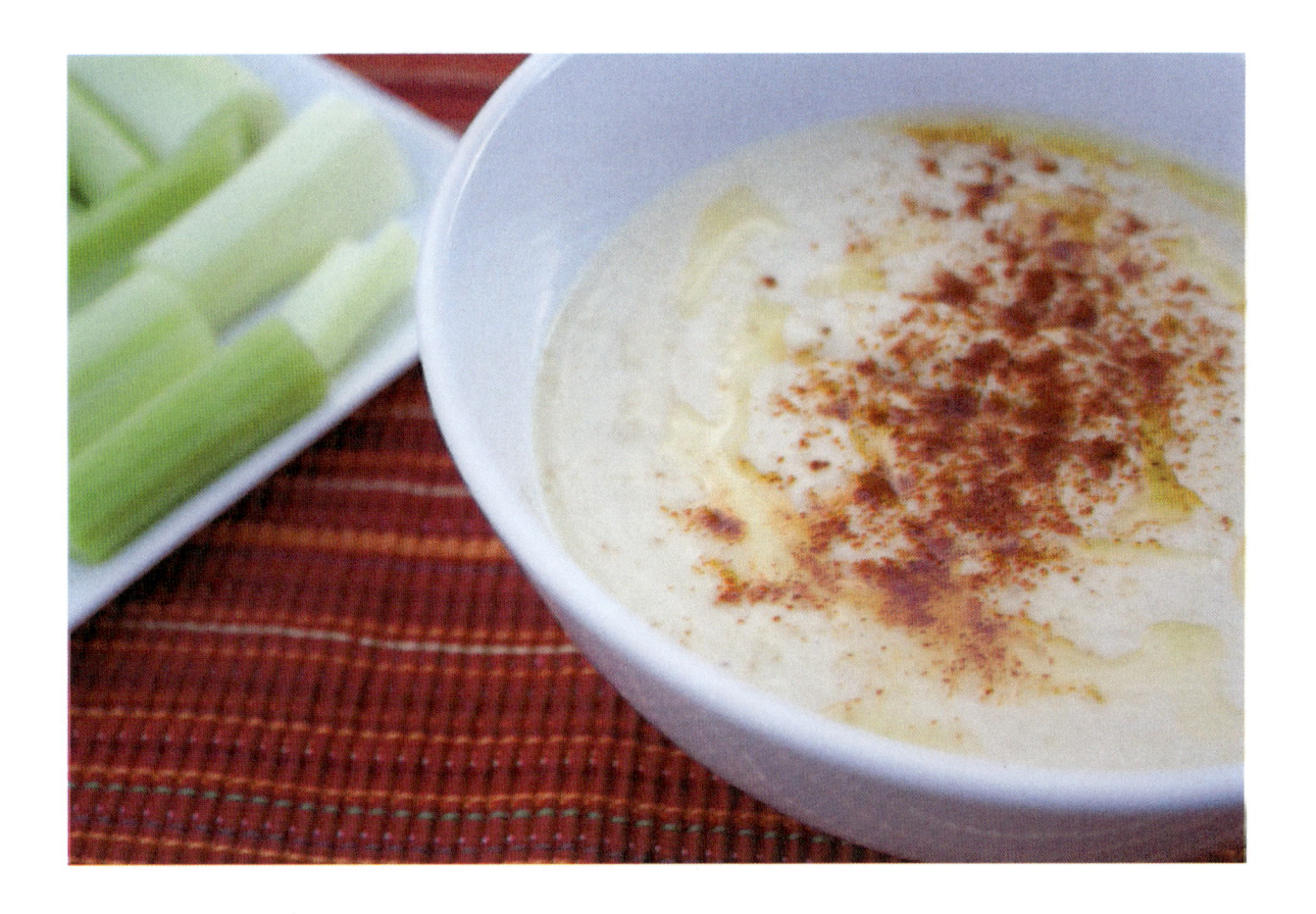

Garlic Humus

Humus is a great vehicle for garlic. Experiment with different recipes using nuts and spices.

Place the following ingredients in a blender and blend until smooth.

Ingredients

- 2 cans of chickpeas, drained rinsed
- ¼ C tahini
- juice of 1 whole lemon
- ¼ C olive oil
- ¼ C water (more water may be added as necessary)
- 6 garlic cloves, peeled
- Himalayan pink sea salt
- dash of cayenne pepper

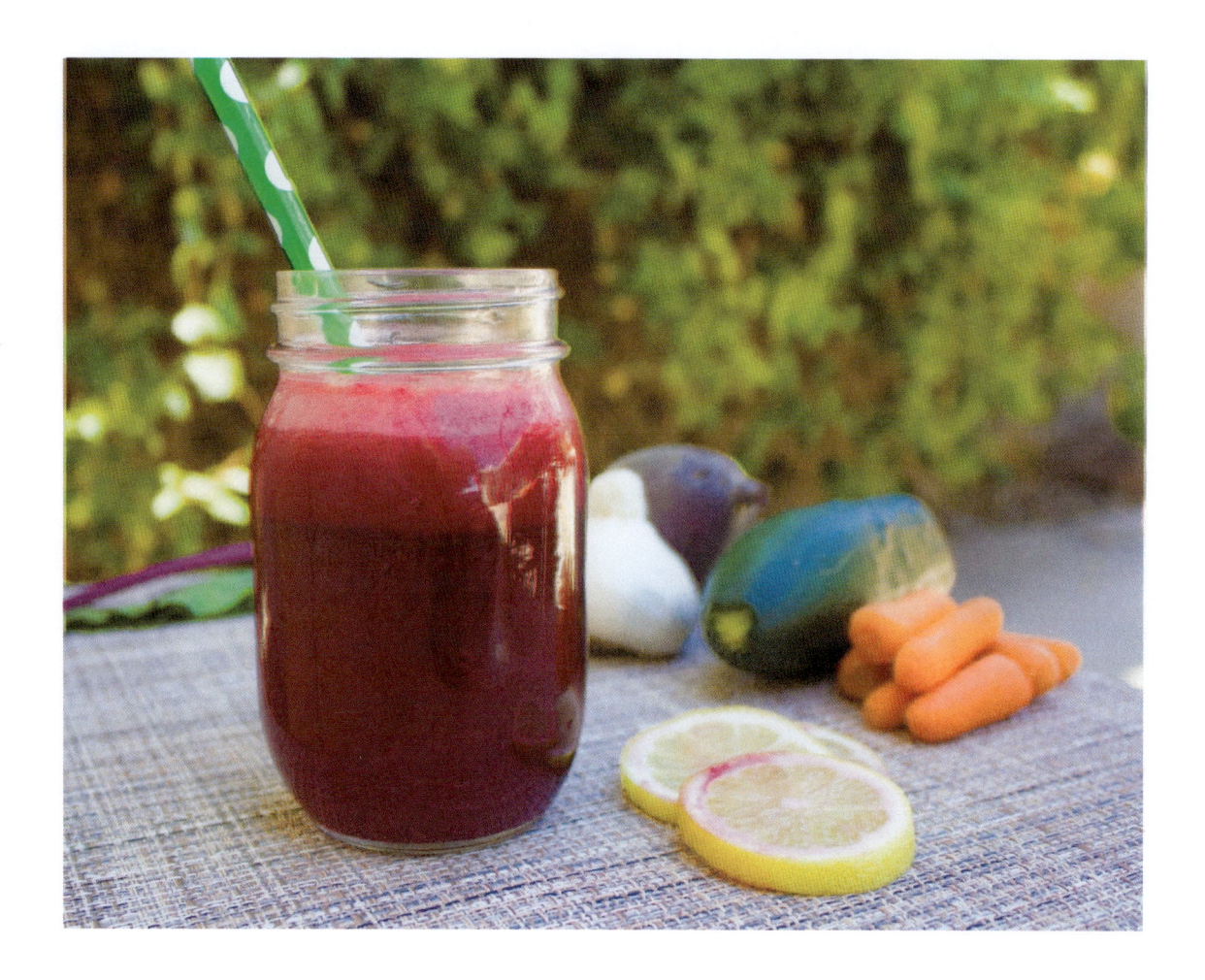

Juice it-Sweet Immune Booster

Make this juice by placing the ingredients into a juicer in the listed order.

Ingredients

Makes about 8 ounces

- 3 carrots chopped
- 1 stalk of celery, chopped
- 1 apple, chopped
- ½ beet, chopped
- ½ cucumber
- 1 C fresh wheat grass
- ¼ C chopped parsley
- I Tbsp lemon
- 2 cloves of garlic

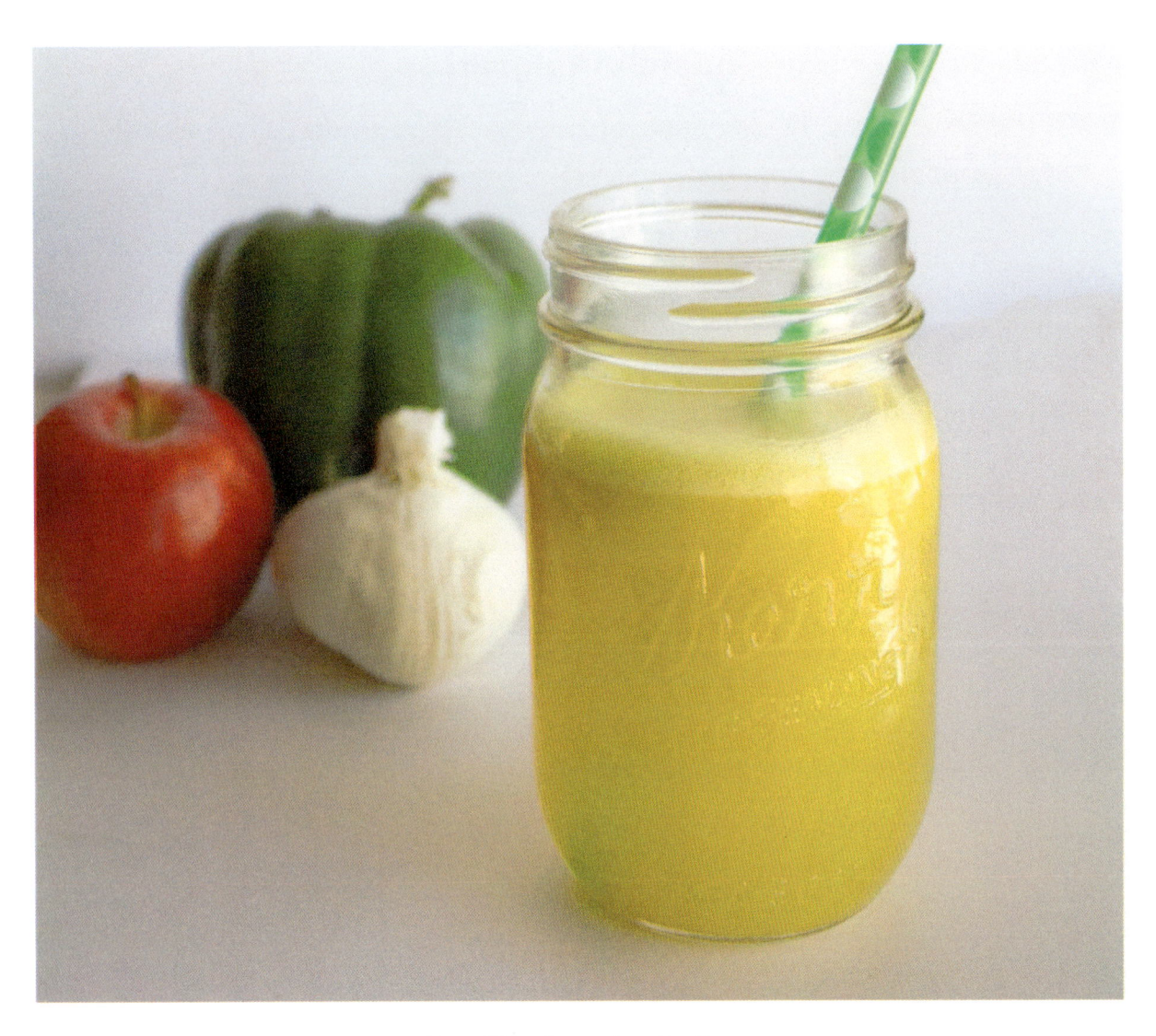

Garlic Apple Juice

Make this juice by placing the ingredients into a juicer in the listed order.

Ingredients

- 1 fresh garlic clove
- 2 granny smith apples, chopped
- 1 bell pepper

Basic Vinaigrette

Ingredients

- ½ C raw apple cider vinegar
- 1 Tbsp Dijon mustard
- 3 medium garlic cloves, minced
- Himalayan sea salt and black pepper
- 1 – 1 ½ C olive oil
- 1 Tbsp honey or maple syrup

Place all ingredients in a mason jar, screw the lid on tightly, and shake. This is a delicious, creamy salad dressing that kids will love. Add parmesan cheese, goat cheese, or walnuts for added zing and flavor.

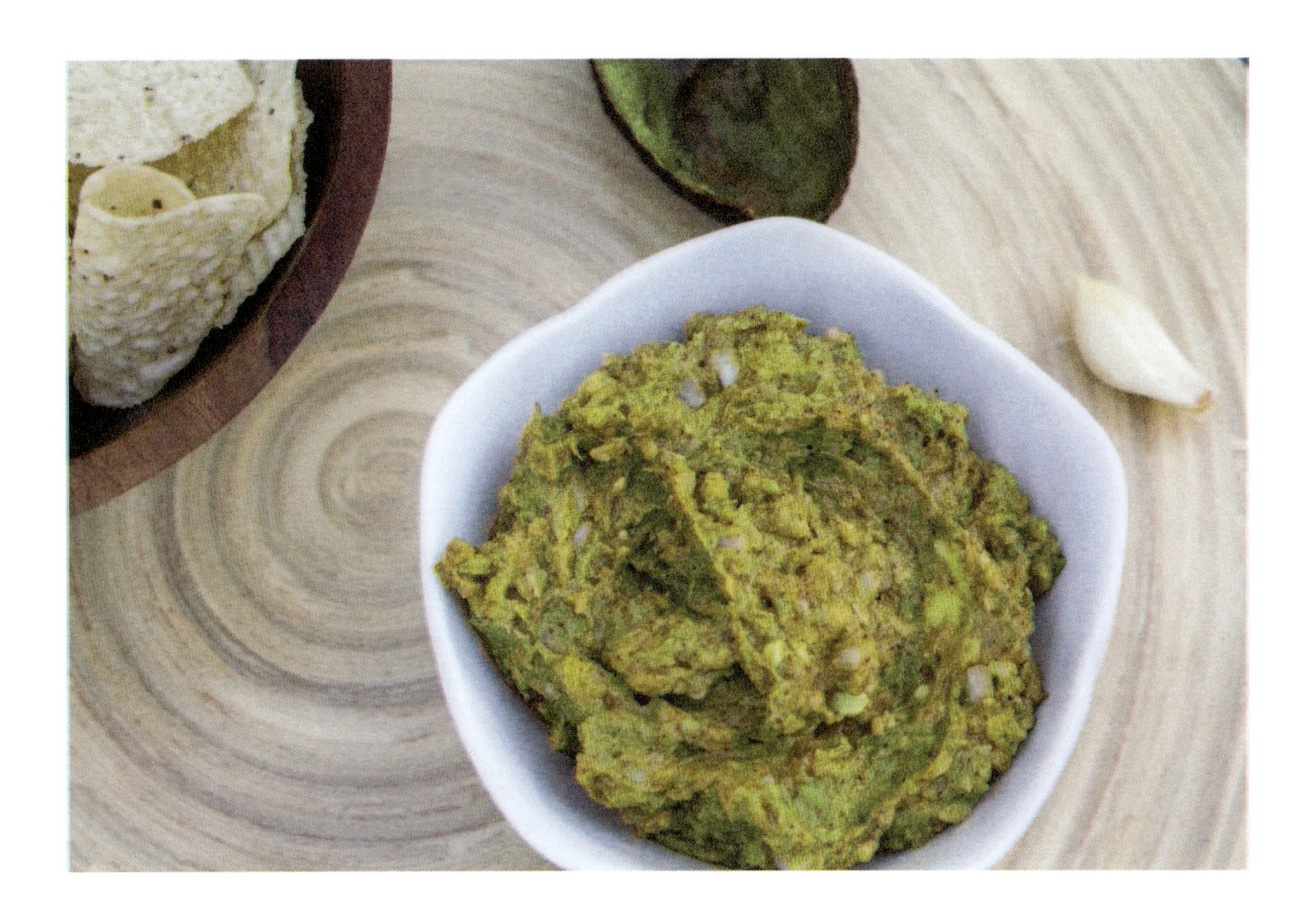

Guacamole

Ingredients

- 3 medium ripe avocados, peeled
- 2 green onions, chopped
- 4 Tbsp crushed garlic
- 3-4 tsp lime juice
- ½ tsp ground cumin
- ½ tsp chili powder
- ½ tsp sea salt

In a bowl, mash the avocados. Add chopped onions, garlic, lime juice, spices, and salt. Serve with tortilla chips made with organic corn.

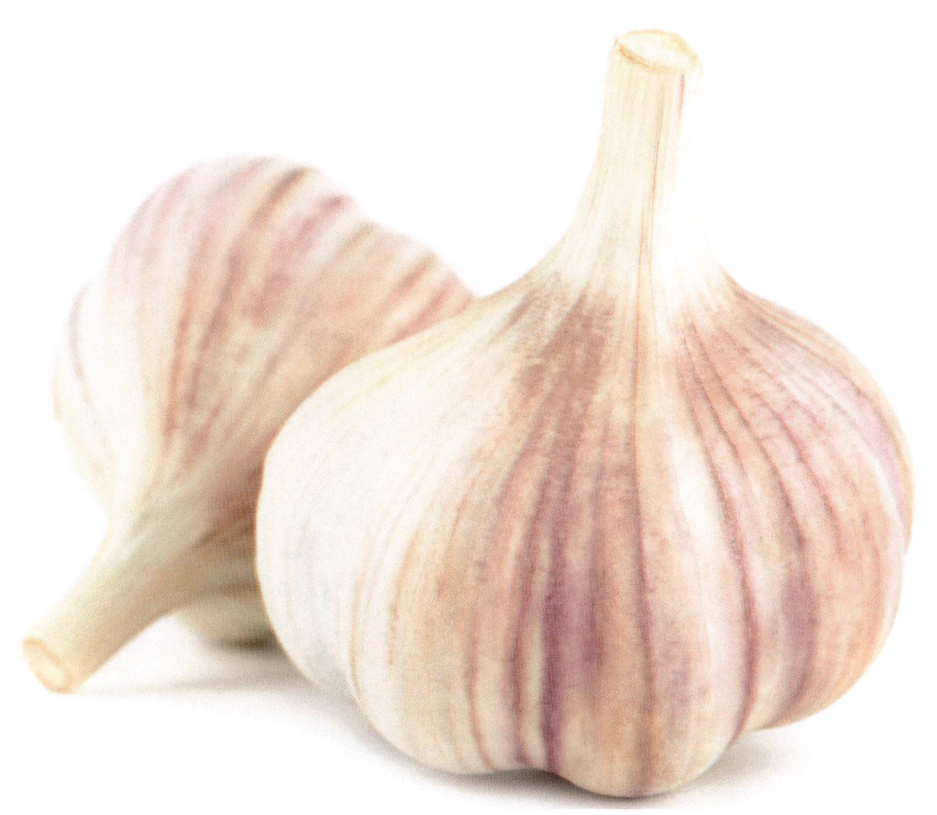

Kitchen Medicine:

Garlic (Allium sativa)

Erin Smith

As an herbalist that also loves to cook, kitchen medicine is second nature for me. I love finding ways to incorporate herbs into food and discovering ways to make medicine that is delicious and multi-functional – one day a medicine, the next adding zing to a favorite dish. Because garlic is so delicious, it's easy to make great medicine that can also be used in the kitchen. The following are some of my favorite simple kitchen medicines. They are great ways to get the medicinal benefits of garlic and can be added to many of your favorite recipes.

You often hear in the natural remedy world that you need to eat your garlic raw to get its medicinal properties. While its true that raw garlic contains the most complete spectrum of garlic's phytochemicals, it is a common misconception that you should just munch on raw garlic cloves. This is really hard on your digestive system. In ancient traditions, garlic was classified as "hot in the fourth degree," which means it is one of the hottest herbs. If you place a cut clove of garlic directly on your skin and leave it there, it will burn the skin, sometimes as badly as a second-degree burn (don't try this!). It's that "hot," so imagine what it does internally if you eat a lot of raw garlic. Daily consumption of straight raw garlic can destroy the mucosal lining of your digestive system. So if you want to get the powerful medicinal properties from raw garlic it is best to eat it in a carrier, such as oil.

Bruschetta

Bruschetta is a classic Italian antipasto made traditionally with olive oil, garlic, fresh tomatoes, and basil. While you might be used to enjoying it at your favorite Italian restaurant, it's also a delicious and easy way to get the medicinal properties of raw garlic. The olive oil and tomato juices help coat the garlic, making it easier for your body to digest while diffusing the heat. Feel free to play around with this recipe and add other vegetables, white beans, different fresh herbs, etc. Add extra garlic to make it even more medicinal. Or if you are in a rush, just add chopped garlic to olive oil and eat with toast or a cracker.

- 3-4 medium tomatoes, seeded and chopped
- 2 cloves of garlic, finely chopped
- 2 Tbsp olive oil
- 6-8 basil leaves, finely chopped
- salt and pepper, to taste

Combine all the ingredients in a bowl and eat by the spoonful or on a cracker or toast. Store in refrigerator. It's best to make in smaller batches; fresh garlic does start to lose its potency the longer it sits.

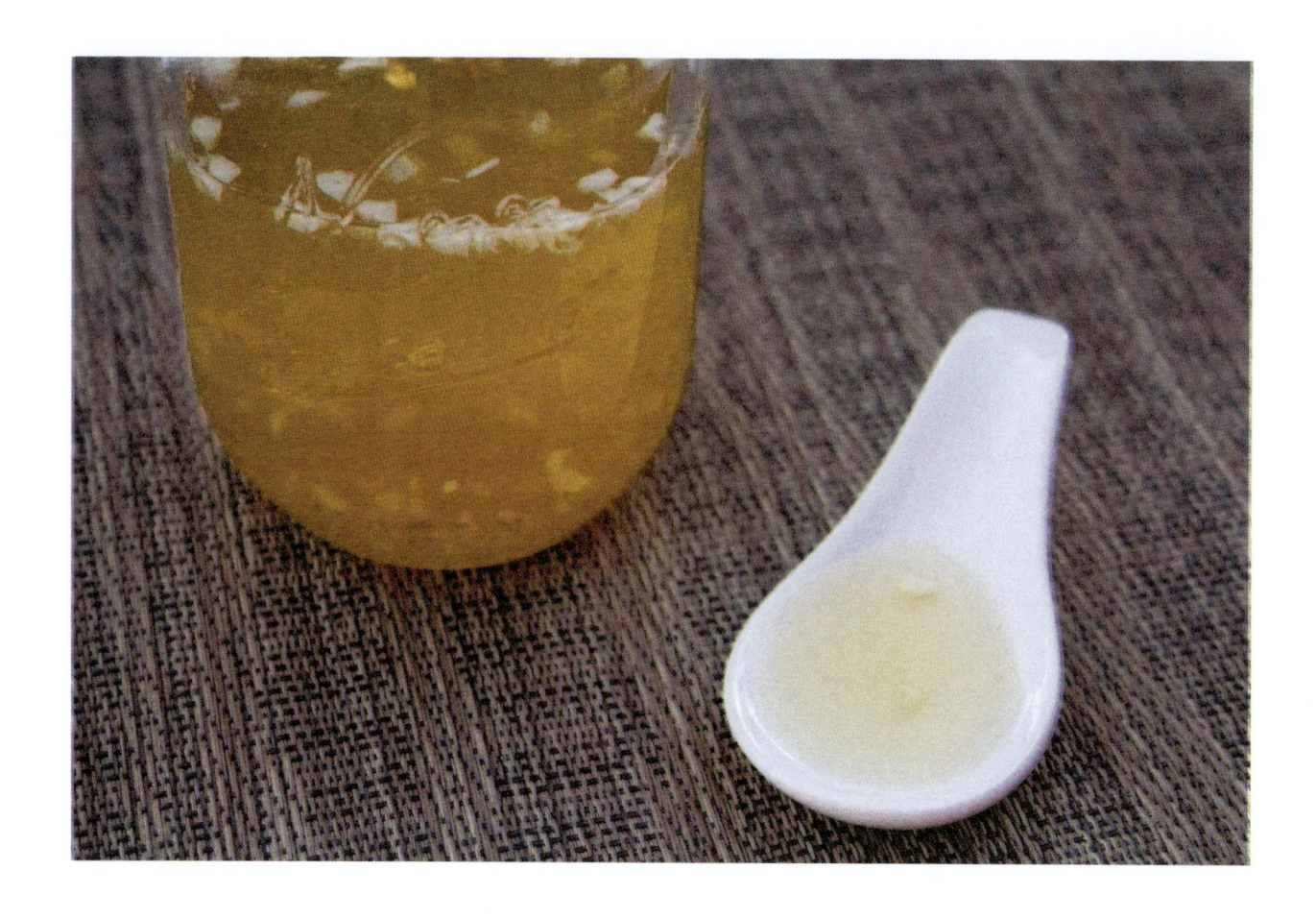

Garlic Vinegar

I tend to make garlic vinegar in a 1:3 or 1:4 ratio (1 part herb to 3 or 4 parts vinegar), but if you want a real kick you can certainly try it at a 1:1 ratio. In general, I make all my herbal vinegars with raw apple cider vinegar, but you can use any vinegar you choose (avoid distilled vinegar). I recommend using the vinegar you use the most and is most versatile.

Ingredients

- 3 heads of organic garlic, peeled and roughly chopped
- raw apple cider vinegar, or vinegar of choice
- glass jar (do not use plastic)

Directions

Place chopped garlic into glass jar and cover with apple cider vinegar until about an inch below the top of the jar. You want to make sure your garlic is completely covered with vinegar. If it floats on the top at first that is fine, as long as it's not sticking up out of the vinegar because this will attract bacteria. As it absorbs the vinegar, the garlic tends to sink to the bottom. Cover with lid and allow to sit for 4-6 weeks. At this point you can strain it or continue to steep and use as needed (once the garlic is sticking out of the vinegar, its best to strain). Use as medicine by the spoonful or to add a kick of garlic to your salad dressings, tuna salad, and other favorite recipes that call for vinegar.

IMPORTANT: Vinegar corrodes metal. Do not let vinegar touch a metal lid or it will ruin your medicine. If you are using a canning jar with a metal lid, cover with plastic wrap or parchment paper first and then put the lid on so that the vinegar does not come into contact with it. You can also purchase plastic lids for this. I often save any glass jars that have plastic lids to reuse for my herbal vinegars.

Garlic Oxymel

Oxy- what?! Yep, this funny name is what you get when you make a vinegar and honey extract. Oxymel is an ancient form of medicine and was commonly used in traditional Greek and Arabic medicine. It's a great way to get the medicinal benefits of garlic. Vinegars are just as effective as alcohol at extracting medicinal compounds from herbs, and they are great for those that are avoiding alcohol. Plus, I love to create herbal vinegars and use them in various recipes, giving your food an extra medicinal kick.

There are number of different ways to make an oxymel and none of them are wrong; it's really just a matter of preference. The honey in oxymels cuts the acidity of the vinegar, making them easier to take in larger quantities.

I like to make my oxymels in a 1:3 ratio (1 part herb to 3 parts vinegar/honey). Many people do vinegar and honey in equal parts, but I prefer mine with less honey. You can play around with it and find the ratio that you like best.

To make an oxymels you have a few options:

1. If you already have garlic vinegar made you can turn it into an oxymel by simply adding honey to your vinegar in your preferred ratio. Start with 1 part honey to 3 parts garlic vinegar. If you prefer it to be a bit sweeter, combine honey and vinegar in equal parts.

2. If you are making an oxymel from scratch, follow the instructions for making garlic vinegar mentioned above. Instead of covering with vinegar, add honey to the jar in the desired amount. Again, I suggest starting small, about 1/3 the amount of vinegar. Add the vinegar. Seal with plastic lid (or plastic wrap and metal lid) and shake vigorously. Allow to sit for 4-6 weeks, shaking daily the first week. When ready, strain and bottle.

3. The third option is to make garlic vinegar and garlic infused honey (see below) and then combine them (1:3, 1:2, or 1:1 ratio) to make an oxymel. Some feel this makes a more potent medicine as both the honey and vinegar have been infused on their own.

Don't stop with garlic, oxymels can be made from any herb. They can be taken by the spoonful as a medicine or you can play around with them in the kitchen. They are regaining popularity in the cocktail world and can also be mixed with sparkling water for a nice, refreshing summer beverage that also happens to be good for you.

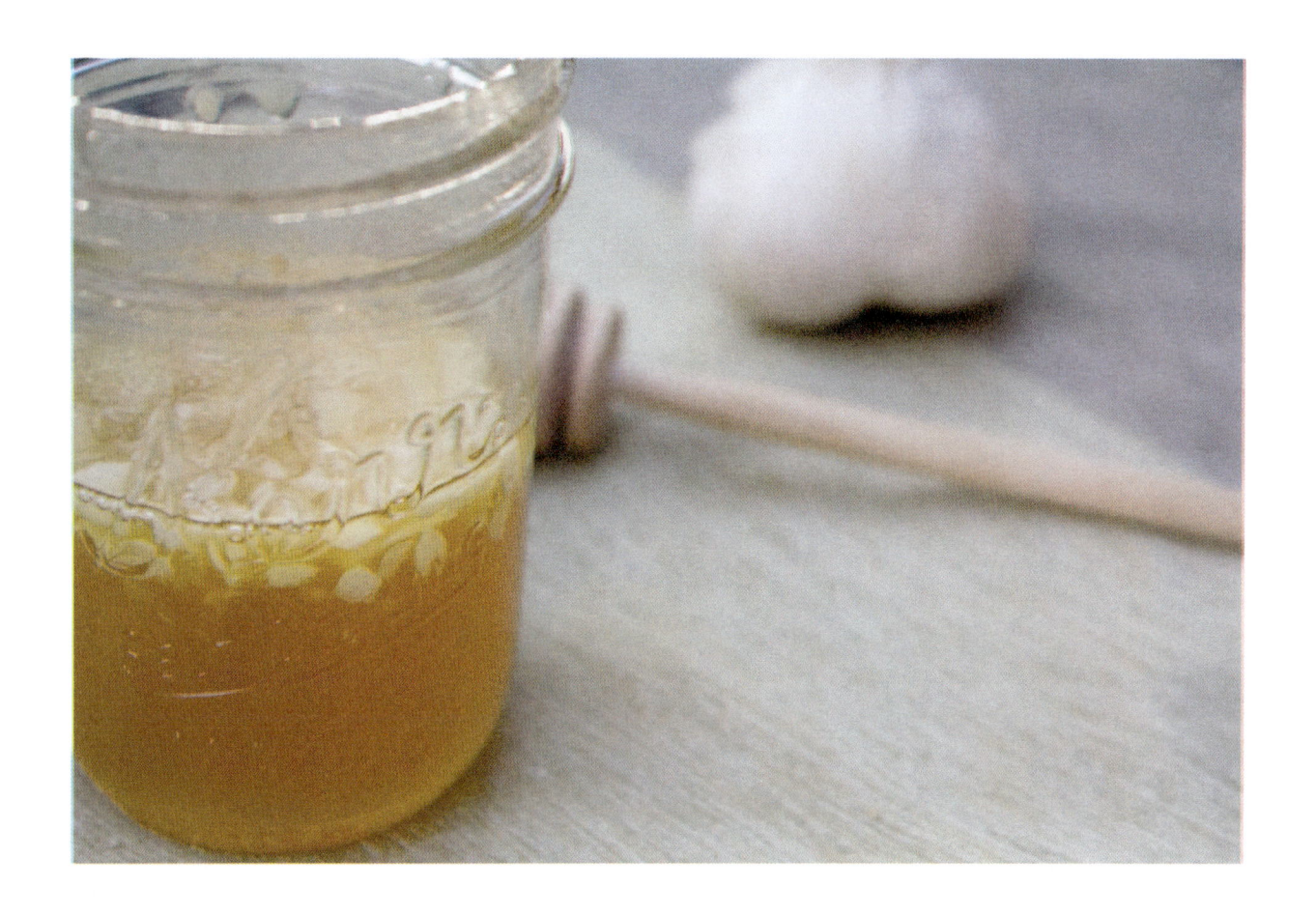

Garlic Infused Honey

Garlic honey is not only great medicine, it's also delicious! You can use this as a way to get garlic's great medicinal properties or as a culinary treat. As a medicine, you can take it straight up by the teaspoonful for sore throats, colds, and flu, or you can dissolve it in a cup of hot water and drink. You can also use it to make syrups, combining with other herbs of your choice. For this, I usually make a decoction of the other herbs and then use garlic honey as the sweetener. Remember that honey is a lot sweeter than sugar, so use less than you would sugar in your syrup recipes.

I prefer to make garlic honey in smaller batches as I think it tastes best when relatively fresh. But if you fall in love with this, you can definitely make it in larger batches. There are no rules for this; the following is just a guideline to get you started. If you prefer it to be more garlicky (and even more of a medicinal powerhouse), fill the jar completely with garlic. If you prefer to make a batch that is more for culinary use, you might use less garlic so that it has a lighter flavor.

Ingredients

- 1 small head of garlic
- 7 oz of raw, local honey

In an 8 oz canning jar, pour in about an inch of the raw honey. Peel all the garlic cloves and crush with the side of a knife. Roughly chop and place into the jar and cover with the remaining honey. Stir with a spoon until all the garlic is coated in honey. Seal with the lid and turn the jar upside down and let stand. After awhile, turn right side up and let stand. Repeat until you feel the garlic is well coated and blended, then allow to steep for a minimum of 3 weeks. I leave the garlic in the honey and allow it to continue to steep while I use it.

If you prefer to be able to remove the garlic pieces, I suggest making it the following way instead:

Place chopped fresh garlic into a "tea pocket," filling the bag but leaving enough space at the top for it to fold over the edge of the jar. Hold the tea pocket to the side of the jar and fill the jar with honey, moving the bag around slightly to ensure that it is completely surrounded by honey. It is important that all the garlic in the tea pocket is under the honey. If you have garlic that is not fully immersed in honey, remove some of the garlic from the bag. With the top part of the pocket sticking out of the jar so that it can be removed later, seal the lid. Allow to steep for 4-6 weeks. When ready, slowly remove the tea bag, gently scraping as much of the honey from the outside of the bag as possible.

One of my favorite ways to use garlic honey in the kitchen is to drizzle it on top of a cracker topped with goat cheese and walnuts. It's as addictive as it sounds!

A Glossary of Herbalism

Nina Katz

Do you feel befuddled by all of those terms? Are you curious about what a menstruum might be, or a nervine? Wondering what the exact difference is between an infusion and a decoction? Or what it means to macerate? Read on; the herbalist lexicographer will reveal it all!

Ad*ap*togen	n.	An herb that enhances one's ability to thrive despite stress. Eleuthero, or Siberian Ginseng *(Eleutherococcus senticosus)* is a well-known adaptogen.
*Ae*rial *parts*	n. pl.	The parts of a plant that grow above ground. Stems, leaves, and flowers are all aerial parts, in contrast to roots and rhizomes.
*Al*terative	n.	An herb that restores the body to health gradually and sustainably by strengthening one or more of the body's systems, such as the digestive or lymphatic system, or one or more of the vital organs, such as the liver or kidneys. Burdock *(Arctium lappa)* is an alterative.
	adj.	Restoring health gradually, as by strengthening one or more of the body's systems or vital organs.
Anthel*min*tic	n.	A substance that eliminates intestinal worms.
Anthel*min*	adj.	Being of or concerning a substance that eliminates intestinal worms.
*An*ti-ca*tar*rhal	n.	A substance that reduces or slows down the production of phlegm.
	adj.	Being of or concerning a substance that reduces or slows down the production of phlegm.
Anti-emetic	n.	A substance that treats nausea. Ginger *(Zingiber officinale)* is anti-emetic.
	adj.	Being of or concerning a substance that treats nausea.
Anti-mic*ro*bial	n.	An herb or a preparation that helps the body fight off microbial infections, whether viral, bacterial, fungal, or parasitic. Herbal anti-microbials may do this by killing the microbes directly, but more often achieve this by enhancing immune function and

		helping the body to fight off disease and restore balance.
	adj.	Being of or concerning an herb or a preparation that helps the body fight off microbial infections.
Aperient	n.	A gentle laxative, such as seaweed, plantain seeds *(Plantago spp.)*, or ripe bananas.
	adj.	Being of or concerning a gentle laxative.
Aphrodisiac	n.	A substance that enhances sexual interest or desire.
	adj.	Being of or relating to a substance that enhances sexual interest or desire.
Astringent	n.	A food, herb, or preparation that causes tissues to constrict, or draw in. Astringents help stop bleeding, diarrhea, and other conditions in which some bodily substance is flowing excessively. Some astringents, such as Wild Plantain *(Plantago major)*, draw so powerfully that they can remove splinters.
	adj	Causing tissues to constrict, and thereby helping to stop excessive loss of body fluids.
Bitter	n.	A food, herb, or preparation that stimulates the liver and digestive organs through its bitter flavor. Dandelion *(Taraxacum officinale)* and Gentian *(Gentiana lutea)* are both bitters. Also called *digestive bitter*.
Carminative	n.	A food, herb, or preparation that reduces the buildup or facilitates the release of intestinal gases. Cardamom *(Amomum spp. and Elettaria spp)* and Fennel *(Foeniculum vulgare)* are carminatives.
	adj.	Characterized as reducing the buildup or facilitating the release of intestinal gases.
Carrier Oil	n.	A non-medicinal oil, such as olive or sesame oil, used to dilute an essential oil.
Catarrh	n.	An inflammation of the mucous membranes resulting in an overproduction of phlegm.
Compound	v.	To create a medicinal formula using two or more components.
	n.	An herbal preparation consisting of two or more

		herbs.
*Com*press	n.	A topical preparation consisting of a cloth soaked in a liquid herbal extract, such as an infusion or decoction, and applied, usually warm or hot, to the body. A washcloth soaked in a hot ginger decoction and applied to a sore muscle is a compress.
De*coct*	v.	To prepare by simmering in water, usually for at least 20 minutes. One usually decocts barks, roots, *rhizomes*, hard seeds, twigs, and nuts.
De*coc*tion	n.	An herbal preparation made by simmering the plant parts in water, usually for at least 20 minutes.
De*mul*cent	n.	An herb with a smooth, slippery texture soothing to the mucous membranes, i.e. the tissues lining the respiratory and digestive tracts. Slippery elm *(Ulmus rubra)*, marshmallow root *(Althaea officinalis)*, and sassafras *(Sassafras albidum, Sassafras officinale)* are all demulcents.
	adj.	Having a smooth, slippery texture that soothes the mucous membranes.
Dipho*re*tic	n.	An herb or preparation that opens the pores of the skin, facilitates sweat, and thereby lowers fevers. In Chinese medicine, diaphoretics are said to "release the exterior." □ Yarrow *(Achillea millefolium)* is a diaphoretic.
	adj.	Opening the pores, facilitating sweat, and thereby lowering fevers.
Di*ges*tive	n.	An herb, food, or preparation that promotes the healthy breakdown, assimilation, and elimination of food, as by gently stimulating the digestive tract in preparation for a meal. Dandelion *(Taraxacum officinale)* and bitter salad greens are digestives.
	adj. 1	Concerning or being part of the bodily system responsible for the breakdown, assimilation, and elimination of food.

	adj. 2	Promoting the healthy breakdown, assimilation, and/or elimination of food.
Diu*r*etic	n.	A substance that facilitates or increases urination. Diuretics can improve kidney function and treat swelling. Excessive use of diuretics can also tax the kidneys. Stinging Nettles *(Urtica dioica)*, cucumbers, and coffee are all diuretics.
	adj.	Facilitating or increasing urination.
Em*men*agogue	n.	An herb or preparation that facilitates or increases menstrual flow. Black cohosh *(Cimicifuga racemosa)* is an emmenagogue. Emmenagogues are generally contraindicated in pregnancy.
	adj.	Facilitating or increasing menstrual flow.
Es*sen*tial *Oil*	n.	An oil characterized by a strong aroma, strong taste, the presence of terpines, and by vaporizing in low temperatures. Essential oils are components of many plants, and when isolated, make fairly strong medicine used primarily externally or for inhalation, and usually not safe for internal use.
	n. 1	A preparation made by chemically removing the soluble parts of a substance into a solvent or menstruum. Herbalists often make extracts using water, alcohol, glycerin, vinegar, oil, or combinations of these. Infusions, medicinal vinegars, tinctures, decoctions, and medicinal oils are all extracts.
	n. 2	A tincture.
Ex*tract*	v.	To remove the soluble parts of a substance into a solvent or menstruum by chemical means.
*Fe*brifuge	n.	An herb or preparation that lowers fevers. Yarrow *(Achillea millefolium)*, ginger *(Zingiber officinale)*, and boneset *(Eupatorium perfoliatum)* are all febrifuges.
Ga*lac*tagogue	n.	A substance that increases the production or flow of milk; a remedy that aids lactation. Nettle *(Urtica dioica)* and hops *(Humulus lupulus)* are galactagogues.
*Glan*dular	n.	A substance that treats the adrenal, thyroid, or other

		glands. Nettle seeds *(Urtica dioica)* are a glandular for the adrenals.
	adj.	Relating to or treating the adrenal, thyroid, or other glands.
He*p*atic	n.	A substance that treats the liver. Dandelion *(Taraxacum officinale)* is a hepatic.
Hyp*n*otic	n.	An herb or preparation that induces sleep. Chamomile *(Matricaria recutita)* and valerian *(Valeriana officinale)* are both hypnotics.
	adj.	Inducing sleep.
In*fu*se	v.	To prepare by steeping in water, especially hot water, straining, and squeezing the marc.
In*fu*sion	n.	A preparation made by first steeping one or more plants or plant parts in water, most often hot water, and then straining the plant material, usually while squeezing the marc. An infusion extracts the flavor, aroma, and water-soluble nutritional and medicinal constituents into the water.
Long In*fu*sion	n.	An infusion that steeps for three or more hours. Long infusions often steep overnight.
Lym*ph*atic	n.	A substance that stimulates the circulation of lymph or *tonifies* the vessels or organs involved in the circulation or storage of lymph.
*M*acerate	v.	To soak a plant or plant parts in a *menstruum* so as to extract the medicinal constituents chemically.
Marc	n.	The plant material left after straining a preparation made by steeping, simmering, or macerating.
Me*n*struum	n.	(Plural, **menstrua** or **menstruums**.) The solvent used to extract the medicinal and/or nutritional constituents from a plant. Water, alcohol, vinegar, and glycerin are among the more common menstrua.
*M*ucilage	n.	A thick, slippery, *demulcent* substance produced by a plant or microorganism.
Muci*lag*inous	n.	Having or producing mucilage; *demulcent.* Okra, marshmallow root *(Althaea officinalis)*, sassafras *(Sassafras albidum, Sassafras officinale)*, and slippery elm *(Ulmus rubra)* are all mucilaginous.
*Ner*vine	n.	An herb or preparation that helps with problems traditionally associated with the nerves, such as mental health issues, insomnia, and pain.

	adj.	Helping with problems traditionally associated with the nerves, such as mental health issues, insomnia, and pain.
Pectoral	n.	A substance that treats the lungs or the respiratory system.
Poultice	n.	A mass of plant material or other substances, usually mashed, gnashed, moistened, or heated, and placed directly on the skin. Sometimes covered by a cloth or adhesive. A plantain *(Plantago spp.)* poultice can draw splinters out.
Rhizome	n.	A usually horizontal stem that grows underground, is marked by nodes from which roots grow down, and branches out to produce a network of new plants growing up from the nodes.
Salve	[sæv] n.	A soothing ointment prepared from beeswax combined with oil, usually medicinal oil, and used in topical applications.
Short Infusion	n.	An *infusion* that steeps for a relatively short period of time, usually 5-30 minutes.
Sedative	n.	A substance that calms and facilitates sleep. Valerian *(Valeriana officinale)* is a sedative.
Sedative	adj.	Calming and facilitating sleep.
Simple	n.	An herbal preparation, such as a tincture or decoction, made from one herb alone.
Simpler	n.	An herbalist who prepares and recommends primarily *simples* rather than compounds.
Spp.	abbr. n.pl.	Species. *Used to indicate more than one species in the same botanical family. Echinacea spp. includes both Echinacea purpurea and Echinacea angustifolium, among other species. Plantago spp. includes both Plantago major and Plantago lanceolata.*
Stimulant	n.	An herb or preparation that increases the activity level in an organ or body system. Echinacea *(Echinacea spp.)* is an immunostimulant; it stimulates the immune system. Cayenne *(Capsicum*

		spp.) is a circulatory stimulant. Rosemary is a stimulant to the nervous, digestive, and circulatory systems.
*Su*dorific	adj.	Increasing sweat or facilitating the release of sweat; cf. *diaphoretic.*
*Sy*rup	n.	A sweet liquid preparation, often made by adding honey or sugar to a decoction.
Tea	n.	A drink made by steeping a plant or plant parts, especially *Camellia sinensis.*
*Ti*sane	n.	An herbal beverage made by decoction or short infusion and not prepared from the tea plant *(Camellia sinensis).*
*Tin*cture	n.	A preparation made by macerating one or more plants or plant parts in a *menstruum,* usually alcohol or glycerin, straining, and squeezing the *marc* in order to extract the chemical constituents into the *menstruum.*
	v.	To prepare by *macerating* in a *menstruum,* straining, and squeezing the marc in order to extract the chemical constituents.
*To*nic	n.	A substance that strengthens one or more organs or systems, or the entire organism. Stinging nettle *(Urtica dioica)* is a general tonic, as well as a specific kidney, liver, and hair tonic. Red raspberry leaf *(Rubus idaeus)* is a reproductive tonic; Mullein *(Verbascum thapsus)* is a respiratory tonic.
*Ton*ify	v.	To strengthen. Nettle *(Urtica dioica)* tonifies the entire body.
Vola*tile* Oil	n.	An oil characterized by volatility, or rapid vaporization at relatively low temperatures; cf. *essential oil.*
Vulnerary	n.	A substance that soothes and heals wounds. Comfrey *(Symphytum officinale)* is an excellent vulnerary.
	adj.	Being or concerning a substance that soothes and heals wounds.

Disclaimer

Nothing provided by Natural Living Mamma LLC, Natural Herbal Living Magazine, or Herb Box should be considered medical advice. Nothing included here is approved by the FDA and the information provided herein is for informational purposes only. Always consult a botanically knowledgeable medical practitioner before starting any course of treatment, especially if you are pregnant, breastfeeding, on any medications, or have any health problems. Natural Living Mamma LLC is not liable for any action or inaction you take based on the information provided here.

Printed in Great Britain
by Amazon